Blood Transfusion Therapy: A Physician's Handbook

Twelfth Edition

2017

To purchase books or to inquire about other book services, including digital downloads and large-quantity sales, please contact our sales department:
- 866.222.2498 (within the United States)
- +1 301.215.6499 (outside the United States)
- +1 301.951.7150 (fax)
- www.aabb.org/marketplace

AABB customer service representatives are available by telephone from 8:30 am to 5:00 pm ET, Monday through Friday, excluding holidays.

Mention of specific products or equipment by contributors to this AABB publication does not represent an endorsement of such products by the AABB nor does it necessarily indicate a preference for those products over other similar competitive products. Any forms and/or procedures in this book are examples. AABB does not imply or guarantee that the materials meet federal, state, or other applicable requirements. It is incumbent on the reader who intends to use any information, forms, policies, or procedures contained in this publication to evaluate such materials for use in light of particular circumstances associated with his or her institution.

The Publisher has made every effort to trace the copyright holders for borrowed material. If any such material has been inadvertently overlooked, the Publisher will be pleased to make the necessary arrangements at the first opportunity. Efforts are made to have publications of the AABB consistent in regard to acceptable practices. However, for several reasons, they may not be. First, as new developments in the practice of blood banking occur, changes may be recommended to the *Standards for Blood Banks and Transfusion Services*. It is not possible, however, to revise each publication at the time such a change is adopted. Thus, it is essential that the most recent edition of the *Standards* be consulted as a reference in regard to current acceptable practices. Second, the views expressed in this publication represent the opinions of authors. The publication of this book does not constitute an endorsement by the AABB of any view expressed herein, and the AABB expressly disclaims any liability arising from any inaccuracy or misstatement.

Editor
Nicholas Bandarenko, MD

Contributing Editors
Sally A. Campbell-Lee, MD
Laura W. Cooling, MD, MSc
Melissa M. Cushing, MD
Meghan Delaney, DO, MPH
Kenneth D. Friedman, MD
Jessica L. Poisson, MD
Jay S. Raval, MD
Mark H. Yazer, MD

Handbook Series Editor
Karen E. King, MD

Other titles in the AABB handbook series:

Hospital Tissue Management: A Practitioner's Handbook, 1st edition
*Edited by A. Brad Eisenbrey, MD, PhD; D. Ted Eastlund, MD;
and Jerome L. Gottschall, MD*

Pediatric Transfusion: A Physician's Handbook, 4th edition
Edited by Edward Wong, MD; Susan D. Roseff, MD; and Karen King, MD

Perioperative Blood Management: A Physician's Handbook, 3rd edition
*Edited by Jonathan H. Waters, MD; Aryeh Shander, MD; and Karen King, MD
(copublished with SABM)*

Therapeutic Apheresis: A Physician's Handbook, 5th edition
Edited by Kendall P. Crookston, MD, PhD, and Karen King, MD

Copyright © 2017 by AABB

*All rights reserved. No part of this book may be
reproduced or transmitted in any form or by any means,
electronic or mechanical, including photocopying,
recording, or by any information storage and retrieval system,
without permission in writing from the Publisher.*

AABB
4550 Montgomery Avenue
Suite 700, North Tower
Bethesda, Maryland 20814-3304

ISBN 978-1-56395-943-1
Printed in the United States

Library of Congress Cataloging-in-Publication Data

Names: Crookston, Kendall P., editor. | Delaney, Meghan, editor. | AABB, issuing body.
Title: Blood transfusion therapy : a physician's handbook / editor, Kendall P. Crookston ; contributing editors, Meghan Delaney [and nine others].
Other titles: Blood transfusion therapy (AABB)
Description: Twelfth edition. | Bethesda, Maryland : AABB, [2017] | Includes bibliographical references and index.
Identifiers: LCCN 2017040022 | ISBN 9781563959431 (alk. paper)
Subjects: | MESH: Blood Transfusion | Handbooks
Classification: LCC RM171 | NLM WB 39 | DDC 615.3/9--dc23
LC record available at https://lccn.loc.gov/2017040022

Contents

Preface ix

1. **BLOOD COMPONENTS** 1

   Concept of Blood Component Therapy 1
   Whole Blood 5
   Red Cell Components 9
   Platelet Components 12
   Granulocytes 17
   Plasma Components........................ 20
   Cryoprecipitated Antihemophilic Factor 24
   Blood Component Modifications.............. 26
   Oxygen Therapeutics 35
   Pathogen Inactivation..................... 36
   References 38

2. **PLASMA DERIVATIVES** 53

   Factor VIII Concentrates 53
   Factor IX Concentrates 61
   Factor X Concentrate....................... 62
   Prothrombin Complex Concentrate 62
   Other Recombinant and Plasma Protein
      Derivatives 63
   Albumin and Plasma Protein Fraction 67
   Synthetic Volume Expanders................. 69
   Immune Globulins 70
   Rh Immune Globulin 72
   References 76

v

3. HEMOSTATIC DISORDERS 81

Overview of Hemostasis..................... 81
Evaluation of Bleeding Disorders............. 85
Platelet Disorders 88
Congenital Bleeding Disorders................ 91
Acquired Bleeding Disorders 110
Prohemostatic Drugs...................... 121
Thrombotic Disorders..................... 123
Disorders of Fibrinolysis 129
References............................... 130

4. TRANSFUSION PRACTICES 141

Surgical Blood Ordering Practices 141
Urgent Transfusion....................... 144
Hematopoietic Progenitor Cell Transplantation.. 145
Solid Organ Transplantation................ 146
Obstetric Transfusion Practices 150
Neonatal Transfusion Practices 153
Pediatric Transfusion Practices.............. 158
Management of Platelet Refractoriness 159
Administration of Blood................... 161
References............................... 165

5. PATIENT BLOOD MANAGEMENT 171

Concept of Patient Blood Management 171
PBM Program Structure 171
Nonsurgical/Preoperative Issues.............. 172
Perioperative Techniques 177
Postoperative Management.................. 184
Blood Utilization Review 186
References............................... 187

6. BLOOD COMPONENT RESUSCITATION IN TRAUMA AND MASSIVE BLEEDING 197

Introduction 197
Hemostatic Resuscitation in Massive Bleeding.. 198
Massive Transfusion Protocol 199
References 211

7. ADVERSE EFFECTS OF BLOOD TRANSFUSION 221

Acute Transfusion Reactions 221
Delayed Hemolytic Transfusion Reactions 238
Hemovigilance.......................... 247
References 248

8. THERAPEUTIC APHERESIS 257

Description............................. 257
Indications 258
Procedural Considerations 265
Complications of Therapeutic Apheresis....... 266
References 269

Index........................... 273

Preface

The goal of *Blood Transfusion Therapy: A Physician's Handbook, 12th edition*, remains the same as when it was first published in 1983: to provide the most current principles of transfusion practice in a readily accessible handbook format. This 12th edition has been updated to be compliant with the 30th edition of *Standards for Blood Banks and Transfusion Services* and harmonized with the 19th edition of the *Technical Manual*. The entire handbook has been extensively reviewed and revised to include the latest recommendations on transfusion medicine practice, based on the most up-to-date scientific evidence. In addition, a new chapter dedicated to massive transfusion has been included.

Chapter 1, Blood Components, contains fast, easy referencing of the major blood products that are currently available in the United States. Details about indications for blood product modifications and special preparation have been updated. This chapter includes additions to available blood products, including a section on pathogen-reduced components.

Chapter 2, Plasma Derivatives, includes descriptions and details related to the available plasma derivatives; the chapter includes useful information on prothrombin complex concentrates and fibrinogen concentrate, as well as a very useful reference table of available derivatives.

Hemostatic disorders are the focus of Chapter 3, organized and written to help readers with this challenging area of transfusion medicine. The chapter contains fundamentals on the management of a variety of important hemostatic disorders with plasma derivatives, pharmaceuticals, and blood products and includes expanded content on anticoagulant drugs, with the latest information on oral direct-acting coagulation inhibitors.

Chapter 4, Transfusion Practices, provides critical, succinctly presented information about transfusion testing, obstetrics, pediatrics, neonates, platelet refractoriness, blood administration, and the transfusion management of hematopoietic stem cell transplant (HSCT) patients. The latter topic is a new section in this chapter. The other content previously found in this *Handbook* regarding HSCT can be found in *Hematopoietic Stem Cell Transplantation: A Handbook for Clinicians, 2nd edition.*

This reorganization was necessary to accommodate the addition of a detailed chapter on Blood Component Resuscitation in Trauma and Massive Bleeding (Chapter 6). The reader will find important up-to-date information on the management of massive transfusion, use of adjuncts, optimizing blood component selection, the resurgence of interest in whole blood, and the multidisciplinary perspectives essential to providing this type of transfusion therapy.

Chapter 5, Patient blood management (PBM) appears for the second time in the *Handbook* series. The chapter highlights salient information about the elements of a successful PBM program; iron supplementation; perioperative issues such as preoperative anemia management, blood recovery, hemodilution, and viscoelastic coagulation monitoring; as well as transfusion guidelines and blood utilization.

Chapter 7, Adverse Effects of Transfusion, has critical information for recognizing, managing, and understanding the mechanism of both acute and delayed complications of transfusion, including TACO and TRALI. The most current risks of transfusion-transmitted diseases are detailed.

The 8th and final chapter in the handbook, Therapeutic Apheresis, has been updated and revised to reflect the 2016 American Society for Apheresis evidence-based guidelines regarding the indications for therapeutic apheresis.

The goal of this handbook is to provide a thorough, yet convenient and concise, reference in an accessible book that will fit in one's lab coat pocket. References have been updated to include the latest literature, facilitating access to more in-depth information, if needed.

The editors would like to thank the many individuals who contributed to this handbook. We wish to express our deep appreciation to Jansen Seheult, MB BCh, MSc for his significant contribution to the Massive Transfusion chapter in working with Mark H. Yazer, MD. We gratefully acknowledge the diligence and hard work of the all contributing editors, who were selected based on both their broad experience in transfusion medicine and their focused expertise in a particular area. Each contributing editor not only performed an intensive revision of the chapter in their area of expertise, but also reviewed the book as a whole. Their expertise and thoroughness are evident in the quality of this handbook. Our final thanks go to Laurie Munk, Jennifer Boyer, Nina Hutchinson, Victoria Barthelmes, and Jay Pennington for their dedication to, and support of, this book and its contributing editors.

Nicholas Bandarenko, MD
Karen E. King, MD
Editors

BLOOD COMPONENTS

Concept of Blood Component Therapy

Blood component therapy refers to the transfusion of the specific part of blood that the patient needs, as opposed to the routine transfusion of Whole Blood (WB). Because one donation of WB can benefit several patients, this practice provides large amounts of a specific blood component to patients who need transfusion and also conserves blood resources. A unit of WB can be processed through a series of centrifugation steps into units of Red Blood Cells (RBCs), Platelets, and Plasma or Cryoprecipitated Antihemophilic Factor (AHF) (see Table 1). Furthermore, the plasma may be used to manufacture several blood derivatives, such as immune globulin, plasma volume expanders, and coagulation factor concentrates, which are then treated to abate or eliminate the risk of virus transmission. (See Chapter 2: Plasma Derivatives.)

Apheresis technology may be used to selectively collect red cells, plasma, and platelets. The volume of each component collected by apheresis from a single donor is at least enough for a single transfusion. Apheresis technology is also capable of collecting 2 RBC units or other combinations of components from a single donor. Thus, the availability of blood components and derivatives permits patients to receive specific hemotherapy that is more targeted than the use of WB.

Because the entire blood collection system is sterile, disposable, and never reused, the risk of donation is similar to that of

Table 1. Commonly Used Blood Components

Component/Product	Composition	Volume	Indications
Whole Blood	Red cells (approx. Hct 40%); plasma; WBCs; platelets	500 mL	Increase both red cell mass and plasma volume (plasma deficient in labile clotting Factors V and VIII)
Red Blood Cells, CPD, CP2D, CPDA-1	Red cells (approx. Hct 65-80%); reduced plasma, WBCs, and platelets	250 mL	Increase red cell mass in symptomatic anemia (WBCs and platelets not functional)
Apheresis RBCs	Red cells (approx. Hct 60%)	300-350 mL	Increase red cell mass in symptomatic anemia
Red Blood Cells, Additive Solution added	Red cells (approx. Hct 60%); reduced plasma, WBCs, and platelets; 100 mL of additive solution	330 mL	Increase red cell mass in symptomatic anemia (WBCs and platelets not functional)
RBCs Leukocytes Reduced (prepared by filtration)	$\geq 85\%$ original volume of red cells; $<5 \times 10^6$ WBCs; few platelets; minimal plasma	225 mL	Increase red cell mass; $<5 \times 10^6$ WBCs to decrease the likelihood of febrile reactions, immunization to leukocytes (HLA antigens), and CMV transmission
Washed RBCs	Red cells (approx. Hct 75%); $<5 \times 10^8$ WBCs; no plasma	180 mL	Increase red cell mass; reduce risk of allergic reactions to plasma proteins

Frozen RBCs; Deglycerolized RBCs	Red cells (approx. Hct 75%); <5 × 10^8 WBCs; no platelets; no plasma	180 mL	Increase red cell mass; minimize febrile or allergic transfusion reactions; use for prolonged RBC storage
Platelet concentrates (Platelets, whole-blood derived)	Platelets (≥5.5 × 10^{10}/unit); red cells; WBCs; plasma	50 mL	Bleeding due to thrombocytopenia or thrombocytopathy
Apheresis Platelets	Platelets (≥3 × 10^{11}/unit); red cells; WBCs; plasma	300 mL	Same as Platelets; may be HLA matched
PAS Platelets	Same as Apheresis Platelets but with 65% of the plasma volume replaced with a sterile buffered solution	300 mL	Repeated allergic transfusion reactions, or 2nd/3rd choice in ABO-mismatched HPC transplantation
Platelets Leukocytes Reduced	Platelets (as above; ≥5.5 × 10^{10}/unit); plasma; <5 × 10^6 WBCs per final dose of Pooled Platelets	300 mL (pooled)	Same as Platelets; <5 × 10^6 WBCs to decrease the likelihood of febrile reactions, alloimmunization to leukocytes (HLA antigens), and CMV transmission
Apheresis Platelets, Leukocytes Reduced	Platelets (>3 × 10^{11}/unit); <5 × 10^6 WBCs/unit; RBCs; plasma	300 mL	Same as Apheresis Platelets; <5 × 10^6 WBCs to decrease the likelihood of febrile reactions, immunization to leukocytes (HLA antigens), and CMV transmission

(Continued)

Table 1. Commonly Used Blood Components (Continued)

Component/Product	Composition	Volume	Indications
FFP; PF24; Thawed Plasma	FFP and PF24: all coagulation factors Thawed Plasma: reduced Factors V and VIII	220 mL	Treatment of some coagulation disorders
Apheresis Granulocytes	Granulocytes ($\geq 1.0 \times 10^{10}$ PMN/unit; may be much greater with G-CSF administration to donor); lymphocytes; platelets ($>2.0 \times 10^{11}$/unit); red cells	220 mL	Provide granulocytes for selected patients with infection and severe neutropenia (<500 PMN/μL)
Cryoprecipitated AHF	Fibrinogen; Factors VIII and XIII; von Willebrand factor; fibronectin	15 mL	Deficiency of fibrinogen or Factor XIII; alternative choice for hemophilia A, von Willebrand disease, and topical fibrin sealant

Hct = hematocrit; WBCs = white blood cells; CPD = citrate-phosphate-dextrose; CP2D = citrate-phosphate dextrose-dextrose; CPDA-1 = citrate-phosphate-dextrose-adenine; RBCs = Red Blood Cells; CMV = cytomegalovirus; PAS = platelet additive solution; HPC = hematopoietic progenitor cell; FFP = Fresh Frozen Plasma; PF24 = Plasma Frozen Within 24 Hours After Phlebotomy; PMN = polymorphonuclear leukocytes; G-CSF = granulocyte colony-stimulating factor; AHF = antihemophilic factor.

any other phlebotomy. The blood collection set (either WB or apheresis collection) is considered a closed system, being open only at the tip of the needle used for donor phlebotomy. When the administration ports of a blood bag have been opened, however, the unit is considered an open system. Components prepared in an open system must be transfused within 24 hours if stored at 1 to 6 C; if stored at 20 to 24 C, components should be transfused within 4 hours to avoid possible bacterial contamination.[1] To prepare components that have the maximal permitted shelf life, integral satellite bags are routinely used to ensure maintenance of the closed system. Alternatively, sterile connection devices permit sterile attachment of separate transfer bags.

Table 1 provides an overview of the different types of blood components available.

Whole Blood

Description

A unit of WB contains approximately 500 mL of blood and 70 mL of anticoagulant-preservative. The hematocrit of a typical unit is 36% to 44%. WB is stored in a monitored refrigerator at 1 to 6 C. The shelf life of WB depends on the preservative used in the blood collection bag; the shelf life of blood in citrate-phosphate-dextrose (CPD) is 21 days, and that of blood collected in CPD-adenine (CPDA-1) is 35 days (see Table 2).

The level of 2,3-diphosphoglycerate (2,3-DPG), a molecule within erythrocytes that facilitates the release of oxygen from hemoglobin, decreases during storage and is regenerated after infusion of the blood.[2] WB stored longer than 24 hours contains few viable platelets or granulocytes. In addition, levels of coagulation Factor V and Factor VIII decrease with storage. However, levels of stable coagulation factors are well-maintained in units of WB during storage.

Table 2. Biochemical Changes in Stored Non-Leukocyte-Reduced Red Blood Cells*

Variable	CPD		CPDA-1				AS-1	AS-3	AS-5
	Whole Blood	Whole Blood	Whole Blood	Whole Blood	Red Blood Cells	Red Blood Cells	Red Blood Cells	Red Blood Cells	Red Blood Cells
Days of storage	0	21	0	35	0	35	42	42	42
% Viable cells (24 hours after transfusion)	100 (64-85)	80	100	79	100	71	76	84	80
pH (measure at 37 C)	7.20	6.84	7.60	6.98	7.55	6.71	6.60	6.50	6.50
ATP (% of initial value)	100	86	100	56 (±16)	100	45 (±12)	60	59	68.50

2,3-DPG (% of initial value)	100	44	100	<10	100	<10	<5	<10	<5
Plasma K+ (mmol/L)	3.90	21.00	4.20	27.30	5.10	78.50†	50.00	46.00	45.60
Plasma	17.00	191.00	82.00	461.00	78.00	658.00†	N/A	386.00	N/A
% Hemolysis	N/A	N/A	N/A	N/A	N/A	N/A	0.50	0.90	0.60

*Reprinted from Roback JD, Grossman BJ, Harris T, Hillyer CD, eds. Technical Manual. 17th ed. Bethesda, MD: AABB, 2011:277.
†Values for plasma hemoglobin and potassium concentrations may appear somewhat high in 35-day-stored Red Blood Cell units; however, the total plasma in these units is only about 70 mL.
2,3-DPG = 2,3-diphosphoglycerate; AS-1 = additive solution formula 1; ATP = adenosine triphosphate; CPD = citrate-phosphate-dextrose; CPDA-1 = citrate-phosphate-dextrose-adenine-1; N/A = not applicable.

Indications

WB provides both oxygen-carrying capacity and blood volume expansion. The primary indication is for treating patients who are actively bleeding and whose anticipated total blood volume loss is >25%. These patients are at risk of developing hemorrhagic shock. The use of WB in massively bleeding patients (those who receive at least 1 blood volume, or more than 10 RBC units, within 24 hours) may limit donor exposures if red cells and plasma would otherwise be given. (See Chapter 6: Blood Component Resuscitation in Trauma and Massive Bleeding.) If a patient is thrombocytopenic, administration of additional platelet components should be considered to provide functional platelets, as the platelets in stored WB become dysfunctional throughout cold storage. Similarly, patients with a clinically significant coagulopathy should be given plasma to replace needed labile and/or depleted coagulation factors.[3]

There is limited justification for the use of "fresh" WB, which is blood collected within the previous 48 hours, in infants undergoing certain complex cardiac surgical procedures.[4] Fresh WB has also been used by the military in the setting of massive transfusion for resuscitation following combat-related injuries.[5-7] Because of the limited indications for the use of WB and the more efficient use of selected blood components, WB has limited availability.[8]

Contraindications and Precautions

Unless a patient requires volume replacement in addition to oxygen-carrying capacity, the use of WB may result in circulatory overload, particularly if rapid infusion is attempted. WB should not be given to patients with chronic anemia who are normovolemic and who require only an increase in oxygen-carrying capacity; RBC units should be given to such patients to decrease the risk of transfusion-associated circulatory overload. (See Chapter 7: Adverse Effects of Blood Transfusion.) Although the red cells in WB have been shown to undergo a variety of ex-vivo changes throughout storage, such as increased potassium levels and mechanical fragility and decreased pH,[9,10] these changes have not correlated with transfusion-related adverse events. However, it is worth mentioning that extracellular potassium levels are highest in longer-stored RBC units, and patients who may be sensitive to potassium infusions, such as neonates or those with kidney failure, may benefit from fresher units in certain cases. Finally, although emerging data suggest that transfusion of WB from low-isohemagglutinin-titer group O donors (with low titers of anti-A and anti-B) are well tolerated without evidence of hemolysis,[11] until definitive studies are performed, WB units should be ABO type-specific to ensure both red cell and plasma compatibility. (See Special Considerations: Use of Cold-Stored Whole Blood, in Chapter 6: Blood Component Resuscitation in Trauma and Massive Bleeding.)

Dose and Administration

In an adult, 1 unit of WB will increase the hemoglobin level by approximately 1 g/dL, or the hematocrit by approximately 3% to 4%. In pediatric patients, a WB transfusion of 8 mL/kg will result in an increase in hemoglobin of approximately 1 g/dL. WB must be administered through a blood administration set containing a 170- to 260-micron filter. The rate of infusion depends on the clinical condition of the patient, but each unit or aliquot should be infused within 4 hours.

Red Cell Components

Description

RBCs are prepared from WB by the removal of 200 to 250 mL of plasma. RBC components may also be collected through apheresis technology, the use of which enables collection of a unit of RBCs and either a second RBC unit or a unit of another blood component. The indications, contraindications, precautions, dosage, and administration of RBC components obtained by apheresis collection (Apheresis Red Blood Cells) are the same as those for RBC components obtained from WB donation.

RBC units are stored at 1 to 6 C in one of several citrate-based anticoagulant-preservative solutions. These solutions contain various amounts and types of preservative agents composed of buffers, dextrose, and possibly adenine.[12] Additive solutions (AS) containing additional agents such as dextrose, adenine, and possibly mannitol may be added to RBCs stored in certain anticoagulant-preservative solutions. The resultant components have different hematocrits and shelf lives. RBCs stored in AS have hematocrits of 55% to 65% and a shelf life of 42 days, whereas those stored in CPDA-1 have hematocrits of 65% to 80% and a shelf life of 35 days.[2,13,14] RBCs stored in CPD have hematocrits similar to those of RBCs stored in CPDA-1 but have a shelf life of only 21 days. RBC components are not a source of functional platelets or granulocytes. RBC components and WB units have the same oxygen-carrying capacity because they contain the same number of red cells.

Indications

Red cells are indicated for treatment of symptomatic anemia in patients who require an increase in oxygen-carrying capacity and red cell mass. The transfusion requirements of each patient should be based on clinical status rather than on any predetermined hematocrit or hemoglobin value.[15,16] AABB guidelines for RBC transfusion are published and available.[17] See Chapter 4: Transfusion Practices.

Contraindications and Precautions

Risks associated with RBC infusion are the same as those encountered with WB. (See also Chapter 7: Adverse Effects of Blood Transfusion.) Although many biochemical and biomechanical changes are known to occur to red cells throughout storage, such as increased fragility, decreased deformability, increased hemolysis, and microparticle generation,[18-21] none of these findings have been definitively correlated with clinical outcomes.[22] Additionally, stored red cells have been implicated in activating the innate immune system, which may lead to an altered inflammatory response and unfavorable effects.[23] However, this hypothesis has also not been definitively confirmed or correlated with clinical outcomes. Upon completion of two randomized trials to address the clinical significance of the red cell storage lesion (the RECESS and ABLE studies), it was found that transfusing fresher-stored RBC units does not impact multiorgan dysfunction scores in complex cardiac surgery patients or critically ill patients.[24,25]

Dose and Administration

In an adult with an average blood volume, 1 RBC unit will increase the hemoglobin level by approximately 1 g/dL or the hematocrit by approximately 3%. In a pediatric patient, RBC transfusion of 10 to 15 mL/kg will raise the hemoglobin level by 2 to 3 g/dL or the hematocrit by approximately 6-9%. RBCs must be transfused through a 170- to 260-micron blood administration filter. Other than isotonic 0.9% normal saline, no solutions or medications should be added to RBCs or infused through the same tubing unless approved for this use by the Food and Drug Administration (FDA).[1] Such approval has been granted for isotonic and isosmotic solutions with 0.9% normal saline, such as Plasma-Lyte A and Normosol, to be infused with RBCs.

The higher hematocrit of CPD or CPDA-1 components results in greater viscosity, which may slow the transfusion rate. The lower hematocrit of RBC units containing AS permits more rapid infusion rates. For patients at risk for circulatory overload and for pediatric patients, concern over the additional volume resulting from the 100 mL of AS may warrant a slower transfusion rate, diuresis in the peritransfusion period, selection of RBC components without AS, or concentrating the component by centrifugation or sedimentation.

Platelet Components

Description

Platelets prepared from individual units of WB by centrifugation have been referred to as "random-donor platelets" or "whole blood-derived platelet concentrates" (herein referred to as PCs). Although units should contain at least 5.5×10^{10} platelets, most units contain more than this amount. PCs should be suspended in sufficient plasma (usually 50 to 70 mL) to maintain a pH greater than 6.2 throughout the storage period.[1]

A platelet unit that is collected from an individual donor during a 1- to 2-hour apheresis procedure (Apheresis Platelets) must contain at least 3×10^{11} platelets,[1] which is equal to 4 to 6 PC units. The volume of plasma in this component varies from 200 to 400 mL. The indications, contraindications, precautions, dosage, and administration of Apheresis Platelets are the same as those for PCs, with the exception that Apheresis Platelets are often preferentially used when the platelets to be transfused must have a specific antigen profile because of platelet refractoriness. (See Management of Platelet Refractoriness in Chapter 4: Transfusion Practices.)

Platelets from any source may be stored in the blood bank for as long as 5 days at 20 to 24 C with constant, gentle agitation. Platelets pooled in an open system expire 4 hours from the time the system is opened. Prepooled PCs have the same outdate as Apheresis Platelets. It has been demonstrated that 5-day-old platelets have nearly normal posttransfusion recovery and survival.[26]

Recently, the FDA approved the use of platelet additive solution (PAS) in Apheresis Platelets. The addition of PAS to these platelets involves 65% of the plasma volume being replaced with this sterile buffered solution containing citrate, phosphate, and acetate. PAS platelets have been shown to have a significantly reduced incidence of allergic transfusion reactions without impacting platelet increases in patients at 12 to 24 hours after transfusion.[27] Thus, indications for PAS platelet transfusion include repeated allergic transfusion reactions or ABO-mismatched hematopoietic progenitor cell (HPC) transplantation where the second or third choice of platelets is used.

Pathogen inactivation of platelets has recently been approved by the FDA, with the use of amotosalen plus ultraviolet A (UVA) light technology. These components, referred to as pathogen-reduced platelets, have been shown to inactivate bacteria species that commonly contaminate platelets, as well as viruses and parasites. Platelets treated with the amotosalen/UVA light phototherapy system can be stored in either plasma or PAS. Patients receiving pathogen-reduced platelets do not demonstrate any difference in mortality, clinically significant bleeding, or severe bleeding.[28] However, the 1- and 24-hour corrected count increment (CCI) is lower with pathogen-reduced platelets, and slightly more frequent transfusions of these risk-reduced platelets may be required. (See Pathogen Inactivation section later in this chapter.)

Indications

Platelets are indicated for treatment of bleeding associated with thrombocytopenia (platelet counts usually <50,000/µL) or for use in patients with functionally abnormal platelets (congenital or acquired disorders; see Chapter 3: Hemostatic Disorders).[29-31] They are also indicated during surgery or before certain invasive procedures in patients who have platelet counts <50,000/µL. Prophylactic transfusion of platelets is common for patients who have platelet counts <5000 to 10,000/µL associated with marrow hypoplasia resulting from chemotherapy, tumor invasion, or primary aplasia.[32-34] This range may be higher for patients with complicating clinical factors.[33] Additionally, platelet transfusions are often included in massive transfusion protocols. In the setting of massive bleeding, improved survival has been observed in patients who received a higher ratio of platelet-to-RBC transfusions.[35,36] AABB guidelines for platelet transfusion are published and available.[37] See also Chapter 4: Transfusion Practices.

Contraindications and Precautions

In patients with rapid platelet destruction, such as idiopathic (immune) thrombocytopenia (ITP) and disseminated intravascular coagulation (DIC), transfusion solely to achieve a platelet increment is not clinically appropriate. Patients with thrombocytopenia secondary to sepsis or hypersplenism may also fail to demonstrate an increment in platelet count. In such patients, platelet transfusion should be used in the presence of active bleeding with clinical monitoring. Platelet transfusions are relatively contraindicated in patients with thrombotic thrombocytopenic purpura (TTP) and heparin-induced thrombocytopenia (HIT), but platelets may be transfused if these patients are bleeding.[38]

Transfusion reactions, including febrile nonhemolytic and allergic reactions, may occur. The treatment of fever should not include antipyretics containing aspirin (acetylsalicylic acid), because aspirin will inhibit platelet function. Rapid infusion of platelets may cause circulatory overload and other complications related to increased intravascular volume.[39] The risk of transfusion-transmitted viral disease from either PCs or Apheresis Platelets is small and similar to the risk associated with any other blood component.

Bacterial contamination of platelets is of special concern because this component is stored at room temperature.[40,41] Required prevention strategies, including the use of diversion pouches and implementation of methods to detect bacterial contamination before components are issued, are not 100% effective, and posttransfusion sepsis remains a concern.[42-44] It has been reported that the contamination rate of PCs ranges from 99 to 965 per million, depending on the method of bacteria testing used, and Apheresis Platelets have a reported contamination rate of 167 per million.[44,45] The most common bacteria species isolated in platelet components are coagulase-negative *Staphylococcus*, *Streptococcus* species, *Staphylococcus aureus*, and *Escherichiae coli*.[46]

PCs may contain up to 0.5 mL of red cells per unit, with as much as 2 to 4 mL per pooled component. Similarly, some Apheresis Platelets may be collected by a technique that allows the component to contain 2 mL or more of red cells per unit. Because of the potential presence of this small amount of red cells in a platelet transfusion, patients who are RhD-negative generally should receive platelets only from a D-negative donor. If D-positive platelets must be transfused to D-negative females of childbearing potential or to children, prevention of D immunization through the use of Rh Immune Globulin should be considered.[47]

Platelets containing ABO-incompatible plasma may be transfused; this is an acceptable practice when ABO-compatible platelets are not available or when HLA-matched platelets are required. Plasma contained in transfused units of ABO-incompatible platelets may cause a positive direct antiglobulin test (DAT) result and, very rarely, hemolysis in the recipient.[48,49] Whenever possible, platelets containing ABO-compatible plasma should be selected. Other approaches include volume reduction, incompatible-plasma volume limitations per 24 hours, screening of donors to identify high-titer ABO antibodies, and use of PAS platelets. Currently, there are no standardized approaches or recommendations for transfusion of platelets containing ABO-incompatible plasma.[50-52]

Dose and Administration

The usual dose for a thrombocytopenic bleeding patient is 1 unit of PCs (at least 5.5×10^{10} platelets) per 10 kg body weight (typically, 4 to 8 units for an adult). The PLADO trial investigated the optimal platelet dose for patients undergoing hematopoietic stem cell transplantation or chemotherapy and receiving prophylactic platelet transfusions for the prevention of bleeding; the specific dose of platelets (between one-half dose and a double dose of platelets) did not affect the incidence of bleeding.[53] However, patients receiving the lower dose did require an increased number of transfusions.

One unit of PCs usually increases the platelet count in a 70-kg adult by 5000/µL. One unit of Apheresis Platelets will usually increase the platelet count of a 70-kg adult by 30,000 to 50,000/µL. In children, 5 to 10 mL/kg will increase the platelet count by 50,000 to 100,000/µL. Repeated failure to achieve hemostasis or the expected increment in platelet count may signify the refractory state.[29,54] Immune refractoriness to platelets is most commonly associated with antibodies to HLA antigens and, rarely, with those to platelet-specific antigens. Clinical refractoriness to platelets is associated with bleeding, amphotericin, splenomegaly, DIC, fever, sepsis, viremia, drugs, veno-occlusive disease, or hematopoietic progenitor cell transplantation.[55] Refractoriness is often suspected on the basis of repeatedly poor clinical response to platelet transfusion and a poor posttransfusion platelet count increment. The CCI may be calculated as follows:

$$CCI = \frac{(\Delta \text{ Platelet Count}) \times BSA \times 10^{11}}{\# \text{ Platelets Transfused}}$$

where Δ Platelet Count = the difference between posttransfusion and pretransfusion platelet count in µL; BSA = body surface area in square meters; and # Platelets Transfused = the total number of platelets infused between the pretransfusion and posttransfusion platelet count measurements. Each unit of PCs contains a minimum of 5.5×10^{10} platelets, and a unit of Apheresis Platelets contains at least 3×10^{11} platelets.

A CCI of >7500 to 10,000 from a peripheral blood sample collected within 1 hour after transfusion or a CCI of >4500 from a sample collected approximately 24 hours after transfusion is considered acceptable and is not indicative of refractoriness.[56,57] Patients who repeatedly have poor clinical or 1-hour CCI responses are more likely to be immune-refractory to platelet transfusion and may pose difficult management problems. (See Management of Platelet Refractoriness in Chapter 4: Transfusion Practices.) Patients who are refractory because of the emergence of HLA or human platelet antigen (HPA) alloantibodies usually require HLA/HPA-matched, HLA/HPA-selected, or crossmatched platelets, although it should be noted that additional time is required to perform testing to characterize antibodies and identify platelet units negative for the cognate antigen(s).[54,58] Patients who have adequate 1-hour CCI responses but poor 24-hour CCI recovery are most likely refractory because of nonimmune etiologies, and they may require more frequent or larger doses of platelets.

Platelets must be administered through a blood administration set with a 170- to 260-micron filter. Testing of platelet units for red cell compatibility is not necessary unless 2 mL or more of red cells are present. Because platelets express ABO antigens, it may be preferable to give platelets that are ABO compatible with the patient's plasma in order to optimize recovery. Likewise, it is preferable to give donor plasma that is compatible with the recipient's red cells, particularly if large amounts are given to recipients with small blood volumes.[48] (See Contraindications and Precautions section above for more on incompatibility.) Depending on the source of platelets and the volume required for a given patient, PCs may be pooled before administration or infused individually. Platelets may be volume reduced to prevent circulatory overload or to diminish the transfusion of ABO-incompatible plasma. PCs should be transfused within 4 hours after pooling. Gamma- or x-ray-irradiated platelets or pathogen-reduced platelets must be selected for patients at risk for transfusion-associated graft-vs-host disease (TA-GVHD) (see Blood Component Modifications section).

Granulocytes

Description

Granulocytes are usually prepared by apheresis collection from a single donor.[59] Each unit contains $\geq 1.0 \times 10^{10}$ granulocytes and various amounts of lymphocytes, platelets, and red cells; the unit is then suspended in 200 to 300 mL of plasma. Hydroxyethyl starch (HES, a red-cell-sedimenting agent) may be used to improve the efficiency of collection. Corticosteroids are routinely administered to the donor to facilitate granulocyte collection. Although not used at all centers, administration of granulocyte colony-stimulating factor (G-CSF) to healthy donors can significantly increase the collection of granulocytes to 4 to 8 × 10^{10} granulocytes/bag.[60,61] Healthy donors who receive G-CSF at doses of 5 to 10 µg/kg may experience side effects such as bone pain, myalgia, arthralgia, nausea, vomiting, or headaches.[60,62] These symptoms generally require no treatment or can be treated successfully with acetaminophen.[62] Fluid retention has been observed in some donors who receive repeated daily doses of corticosteroids and G-CSF. Long-term follow-up of volunteer granulocyte donors suggests that G-CSF/dexamethasone stimulation appears to be safe.[63] Granulocytes collected from G-CSF-stimulated donors appear to function normally, although they differ phenotypically from granulocytes collected from unstimulated donors, with increased expression of adhesion molecules.[60]

Transfusion of G-CSF-mobilized granulocyte components typically results in measurable increases in peripheral blood granulocyte counts of 1000/µL or more, which are sustained above baseline for 1 to 2 days.[64] The presence of platelets in granulocyte concentrates is often beneficial because many neutropenic patients are also thrombocytopenic.[64] Granulocytes should be transfused as soon as possible, but they may be stored at 20 to 24 C for up to 24 hours after collection.[65,66]

Indications

The decision to use granulocytes should be made in consultation with the transfusion service physician. The patient typically has neutropenia (neutrophil count <500/µL), bacterial or fungal infection (preferably documented) for 24 to 48 hours, lack of responsiveness to appropriate antimicrobials or other modes of therapy, marrow showing myeloid hypoplasia, and a reasonable chance for recovery of marrow function. Granulocyte transfusions may also be beneficial for neonatal patients with sepsis,[67] neutropenic recipients of abdominal organ transplants with active infections,[68] and patients with hereditary neutrophil function defects such as chronic granulomatous disease. Randomized studies have suggested that granulocyte transfusions of at least 1×10^{10} per transfusion could be beneficial in selected neutropenic patients.[69-72]

It has been suggested that clinical response to granulocyte transfusion therapy may be limited by the dose of granulocytes administered, and it is possible that the larger doses obtained with G-CSF-stimulated donors may lead to enhanced therapeutic benefit. Randomized clinical studies with G-CSF-enhanced doses of granulocytes are needed to define the clinical indications and efficacy of this therapy.[70] Furthermore, the benefit of granulocyte therapy, regardless of dose, has been questioned. A Phase III randomized controlled trial sponsored by the National Institutes of Health [the Resolving Infections in Neutropenia with Granulocytes (RING) Study] evaluated the efficacy of G-CSF/dexamethasone-mobilized granulocyte transfusions in neutropenic patients who received HPC transplantation and/or aggressive chemotherapy with probable or proven infections, using a compositive outcome of survival and microbial response.[73] The results of the trial demonstrated no significant differences between granulocyte transfusion versus control arms, but enrollment was low and a possible treatment effect may have been missed.

Contraindications and Precautions

Successful treatment of the infected neutropenic patient includes appropriate antimicrobial therapy and/or the use of hematopoietic growth factors, in addition to possible use of granulocyte transfusions. If recovery of marrow function is doubtful, granulocyte transfusions are unlikely to alter the ultimate clinical course of a neutropenic patient. Patients who are HLA alloimmunized may be less likely to benefit from random-donor granulocytes.[74] Chills, fever, and allergic reactions may occur and are minimized by slow infusion rates, diphenhydramine and/or meperidine, steroids, and/or nonaspirin antipyretics. In some patients, severe febrile and pulmonary reactions to Apheresis Granulocytes may preclude their further use. There is a risk of viral disease transmission, especially cytomegalovirus (CMV). Thus, CMV-seronegative patients who are at high risk for CMV disease, such as patients undergoing allogeneic progenitor cell transplantation, should receive CMV-seronegative granulocytes. Unlike leukocyte reduction for RBCs and platelets, leukocyte reduction to provide a CMV-safe granulocyte product should not be performed. Immunization to HLA and red cell antigens may occur as well.[75] Gamma or x-ray irradiation should be performed to prevent TA-GVHD. The dose of radiation used to prevent TA-GVHD does not impair the function of granulocytes.

Dose and Administration

Although most blood centers do not perform HLA typing on Apheresis Granulocytes, red cell compatibility testing must be performed because of the large number of red cells present. Single daily granulocyte transfusions are often given, but the kinetics of transfused granulocytes from G-CSF-stimulated donors may allow for every-other-day transfusion.[64] A blood administration set with a 170- to 260-micron filter must be used.

Plasma Components

Description

Several plasma alternatives can be used for coagulation factor replacement, including Fresh Frozen Plasma (FFP), Plasma Frozen Within 24 Hours After Phlebotomy (PF24), and Thawed Plasma. FFP is prepared from WB by separating and freezing the plasma at ≤ -18 C within 8 hours of phlebotomy, if collected in CPD, citrate-phosphate-dextrose-dextrose (CP2D), or CPDA-1.

FFP may also be obtained by apheresis collection. Apheresis technology allows for the collection of the equivalent of 2 units of plasma during a single donation. PF24 is prepared from WB by separating and freezing the plasma at ≤ -18 C within 24 hours of phlebotomy. Except for Factor VIII, PF24 contains similar levels of coagulation factors and inhibitors as FFP. Despite a variable reduction in Factor VIII, the Factor VIII levels in PF24 are generally within the normal range of human plasma.[76,77] Plasma may be stored for as long as 1 year at −18 C or colder. The volume of a typical unit is 200 to 250 mL. Under these conditions, the loss of Factors V and VIII, the labile clotting factors, is minimal. One mL of FFP contains approximately 1 unit of coagulation factor activity.

Recently, the FDA approved the use of two pathogen-reduced plasma products: one uses solvent/detergent treatment and is called Octaplas (OctaPharma AG, Lachen, Switzerland), and the other uses amotosalen plus UVA light, a system identical to that used with platelets. (See Pathogen Inactivation section.)

Once thawed, FFP or PF24 must be stored at 1 to 6 C and transfused within 24 hours. When thawed FFP or PF24 is relabeled as Thawed Plasma, it can be stored for up to 4 additional days. The levels of Factor VIII and Factor V decline during storage, although the latter does not decrease below the hemostatic level of 35%.[78,79] Studies have shown that Thawed Plasma prepared from FFP and that from PF24 have comparable levels of coagulation activities.[77,80] Octaplas must be used within 8 hours if kept at 20 to 25 C, or 24 hours at 2 to 4 C.

Indications

Plasma is indicated for use in bleeding patients or patients undergoing an invasive procedure with multiple coagulation factor deficiencies, such as those secondary to liver disease, DIC, and the dilutional coagulopathy resulting from massive blood component transfusion or volume replacement. Although these are common indications for plasma transfusion, the level of coagulopathy requiring replacement is controversial.[30,81,82] Plasma transfusion can be used for the rapid reversal of warfarin effect in a bleeding patient or in the setting of emergency surgery; however, a more practical approach now implements the initial use of prothrombin complex concentrates. (See Chapter 2: Plasma Derivatives; Chapter 3: Hemostatic Disorders.) Because minor prolongations in coagulation tests are not predictive of excessive bleeding, the prothrombin time (PT) or activated partial thromboplastin time (aPTT) should be indicative of factor levels of 30% or lower, or the international normalized ratio (INR) should be 2.0 or higher, before plasma is used prophylactically.[30,81,83-85]

Plasma is indicated in patients with congenital factor deficiencies for which there is no coagulation concentrate available, such as deficiencies of Factor V or XI. Plasma may also be used as primary therapy and as the principal replacement solution in therapeutic plasma exchange procedures for the treatment of diseases such as TTP and vasculitis-associated diffuse alveolar hemorrhage, or when therapeutic plasma exchange is to be performed proximal to biopsy or surgery. (See Chapter 8: Therapeutic Apheresis.) Plasma Cryoprecipitate Reduced, a plasma component with decreased von Willebrand factor, has also been employed as a replacement solution during therapeutic plasma exchange of patients with TTP, because of the decreased concentration of unusually large von Willebrand factor multimers present in this component.[86,87] Octaplas has been FDA approved for use in patients with acquired multiple coagulation factor deficiency or as a replacement fluid for therapeutic plasma exchange in the treatment of TTP patients; this latter indication is based on a rationale similar to Plasma Cryoprecipitate Reduced in that the solvent/detergent treatment process decreases concentrations of unusually large von Willebrand factor. However, it should be noted that no data support the use of either of these alternative components preferentially.

Contraindications and Precautions

Plasma should not be used to provide intravascular volume expansion, because it exposes patients unnecessarily to the attendant risks of transfusion-transmitted diseases. Albumin, plasma protein fraction, or other colloid or crystalloid solutions that do not transmit infection are safer components to use for intravascular volume expansion. Similarly, plasma should not be used as a source of protein in nutritionally deficient patients. In general, plasma has a risk of infectious disease transmission equal to that of WB. Certain viruses, such as CMV and human T-cell lymphotropic virus, type I, do not appear to be transmitted by plasma because they are associated exclusively with leukocytes.[88] Pathogen inactivation with the amotosalen/UVA light system can be applied to plasma before freezing to markedly reduce the risk of transfusion-transmitted diseases. (See Pathogen Inactivation section.)

Allergic reactions can occur with plasma infusion.[89] IgA-deficient patients at risk for anaphylaxis should receive IgA-deficient plasma.

Plasma products have been associated with transfusion-related acute lung injury (TRALI), now the most frequent cause of transfusion-related fatalities,[90] prompting strategies to reduce this risk. (See Chapter 7: Adverse Effects of Blood Transfusion.)[91] As with transfusion of other blood components, volume overload can occur with plasma infusion.[92]

Dose and Administration

The appropriate dose of plasma depends on the clinical situation and the underlying disease process. When plasma is given for coagulation factor replacement, the dose is 10 to 20 mL/kg (equivalent to 3 to 6 units in an adult). This dose would be expected to increase the level of coagulation factors by 20% immediately after infusion. Plasma is one of the components given to patients with vitamin K deficiency when it is not possible to wait for administered vitamin K to take effect, and when prothrombin complex concentrates are not available. Posttransfusion assessment of the patient's coagulation status is important, and monitoring of coagulation function with clinical assessment, PT, aPTT, or specific factor assays is critical. (See Chapter 3: Hemostatic

Disorders.) As with all blood components, plasma must be given through a standard 170- to 260-micron filter. After thawing, FFP, PF24, and Thawed Plasma should be stored at 1 to 6 C. Compatibility testing is not required, but ABO-compatible plasma is preferred.

Cryoprecipitated Antihemophilic Factor

Description

Cryoprecipitated AHF is a concentrated source of Factor VIII:C (the procoagulant factor), Factor VIII:vWF (von Willebrand factor), fibrinogen, fibronectin, and Factor XIII. It is prepared by thawing 1 unit of FFP at 1 to 6 C. After it is thawed, the supernatant plasma is removed, which leaves the cold-precipitated protein, along with 10 to 15 mL of plasma, in the bag. This material is then refrozen at −18 C or colder within 1 hour and has a shelf life of 1 year. Each bag of Cryoprecipitated AHF contains approximately 80 to 120 units of Factor VIII, at least 150 mg of fibrinogen,[1] approximately 20% to 30% of the Factor XIII present in the initial unit, and approximately 40% to 70% of the von Willebrand factor present in the initial unit. Cryoprecipitated AHF is the main source of concentrated fibrinogen in the United States for the treatment of patients with acquired fibrinogen deficiency.

Indications

Cryoprecipitated AHF may be indicated for the treatment of congenital or acquired fibrinogen deficiency. Although the FDA recently approved a plasma-derived fibrinogen concentrate product for the treatment of bleeding in patients with congenital fibrinogen deficiency, institutions may not routinely maintain the product in inventory.[93] Cryoprecipitated AHF is not indicated in hemophilia A, von Willebrand disease, or Factor XIII deficiency when factor concentrates are available. (See Chapter 2: Plasma Derivatives.) Because it does not contain clinically significant amounts of other coagulation factors, Cryoprecipitated AHF is not indicated as the sole treatment for DIC, but it is an important component in the treatment of disorders with hypofibrinogenemia. Cryoprecipitated AHF has also been reported to be beneficial in treating the bleeding tendency associated with uremia[94]; however, its use should be restricted to those who are unresponsive to nontransfusion therapies, such as dialysis or desmopressin, as these approaches are free of the potential infectious complications of blood components.[95] The use of Cryoprecipitated AHF as a fibrin sealant has largely been replaced by the use of commercially available products. (See Chapter 2: Plasma Derivatives.)[96]

Contraindications and Precautions

Cryoprecipitated AHF should not be used to treat patients with deficiencies of factors other than fibrinogen. It should be used as second-line therapy for hemophilia A, von Willebrand disease, or Factor XIII deficiency when factor concentrates are unavailable. ABO-compatible cryoprecipitate is not required because of the small amount of plasma in this blood component, although that volume of plasma may be clinically significant in infants. In rare instances, infusion of large numbers of ABO-incompatible units of Cryoprecipitated AHF can cause hemolysis, and a positive DAT can be seen with infusion of smaller doses. The risk of infectious disease transmission via Cryoprecipitated AHF is the same as that via plasma.

Dose and Administration

Before infusion, the cryoprecipitate is thawed at 30 to 37 C. Each unit will increase fibrinogen by 5 to 10 mg/dL in an average-size adult. In a child, dosing 1 to 2 units/10 kg will increase fibrinogen levels by up to 100 mg/dL. In a bleeding patient, a reasonable target level for fibrinogen is 100 to 150 mg/dL. (See Chapter 3: Hemostatic Disorders.) Cryoprecipitated AHF is administered through a blood administration set with a 170- to 260-micron filter, and no compatibility testing is required. If Cryoprecipitated AHF from a single donor, a dose pooled from multiple donors before freezing, or a dose pooled from multiple donors using an FDA-approved sterile pooling system is thawed but not used immediately, it may be stored no more than 6 hours at room temperature. If pooled using a non-FDA-approved sterile connecting system, Cryoprecipitated AHF must be transfused within 4 hours after pooling.

Blood Component Modifications

A variety of manipulations can be performed on blood components in the blood bank for patients who would benefit from these modifications. The time frame for these processes can range from minutes to hours, so clear communication with the blood bank is critical for the timely and appropriate allocation of blood components with these unique characteristics. When in doubt, a discussion with the transfusion service physician is advised to optimize the selection of blood component manipulations.

LEUKOCYTE REDUCTION

Description of Modification

All cellular blood components contain leukocytes. RBC units contain 1 to 3×10^9 leukocytes,[97,98] and PCs manufactured from WB contain 0.5 to 1×10^8 leukocytes. These leukocytes are not removed by the standard 170- to 260-micron blood filter.[99-101] Leukocyte-reduced blood components may also be referred to as "filtered" or "CMV safe." While it is required in several countries, universal leukocyte reduction of cellular blood components has been implemented voluntarily by many blood centers in the United States.

AABB *Standards for Blood Banks and Transfusion Services* specifies that RBCs prepared from WB that undergo further modification by leukocyte reduction (Red Blood Cells Leukocytes Reduced) must contain <5 × 10^6 leukocytes and retain at least 85% of the original red cells.[1] Similarly, for Apheresis RBC units that are leukocyte reduced (Apheresis Red Blood Cells Leukocytes Reduced), <5 × 10^6 leukocytes and ≥51 g hemoglobin must be present.[1] PCs that are leukocyte reduced (Platelets Leukocytes Reduced) should contain <8.3 × 10^5 leukocytes per unit and, when pooled (Pooled Platelets Leukocytes Reduced), a final count of <5 × 10^6 leukocytes.[1] Similarly, Apheresis Platelets Leukocytes Reduced must contain <5 × 10^6 leukocytes. The passage of platelets through leukocyte-reduction filters generally removes fewer than 10% of the platelets in the component.[100,101] The newest-generation filters have the ability to efficiently reduce leukocytes in cellular blood components well below the 5 × 10^6 threshold. Storage conditions and durations for leukocyte-reduced RBC or platelet components are the same as that for non-leukocyte-reduced components.

Leukocyte reduction is best achieved by filtration of the unit in the blood center shortly after blood collection (prestorage filtration) or in the transfusion service laboratory before blood issue (laboratory filtration). Leukocyte reduction may be performed at the time of transfusion by passing the blood through one of several commercially available bedside blood filters. Prestorage and laboratory filtration have several advantages over bedside filtration. These methods are generally more effective than bedside filtration, as they more consistently leave <10^6 leukocytes/unit. Additionally, prestorage and laboratory filtration can provide an immediately available inventory of leukocyte-reduced components with a normal shelf life and permit better quality control of residual leukocyte content.[102,103] Prestorage leukocyte reduction is the optimal method of leukocyte reduction because it also results in lower levels of ex-vivo cytokine generation in blood bags during storage and a subsequently lower risk of febrile nonhemolytic transfusion reactions.[104-108] Many apheresis technologies are able to produce leukocyte-reduced components at the time of collection that have the same advantages as prestorage leukocyte-reduced components.[109,110] Bedside filtration usually leaves <5 × 10^6 leukocytes in the transfused blood[111]; however, the success of this method depends on the duration of unit storage, the initial leukocyte content of the unit, and proper use of the leukocyte-reduction filter. Some bedside leukocyte-reduction filters have been associated with hypotension and other adverse effects. Because of the quality-control issues, bedside filtration is not the preferred method of leukocyte reduction and is rarely used.

Indications

Leukocyte-reduced blood components are indicated for 1) use in patients who have had repeated febrile reactions in association with the transfusion of red cells or platelets, 2) prophylaxis against HLA alloimmunization for patients in whom intensive, long-term hemotherapy or organ transplantation is anticipated, and 3) decreasing the risk of transfusion-transmitted CMV.[103] Patients who have received frequent transfusions, and females who have had multiple pregnancies, may become alloimmunized to leukocyte antigens. Consequences of alloimmunization can manifest as febrile transfusion reactions associated with red cell transfusions or as refractoriness to platelet transfusion.[112] With regard to transfusion, allogeneic leukocytes are responsible for the development of antibodies against foreign HLA antigens,[113,114] and the interactions of these recipient antibodies with donor leukocytes are responsible for many recurrent febrile nonhemolytic transfusion reactions after non-leukocyte-reduced red cell component transfusions.[115] Leukocyte reduction of red cell components has been shown to decrease the subsequent incidence of these reactions.[108] For platelet components, clinical studies have demonstrated that febrile nonhemolytic transfusion reactions are associated with transfusion of platelets that have been stored for several days.[116-118] These reactions are caused, in part, by the infusion of pyrogenic cytokines. (See Chapter 7: Adverse Effects of Blood Transfusion.)

With regard to transfusing leukocyte-reduced platelet components for the prevention of febrile reactions in patients who are already alloimmunized against foreign HLA antigens, although the occurrence of febrile reactions may decrease, the use of these components will not improve the low CCI. Obtaining an adequate platelet increment in such patients nearly always requires the use of HLA-matched, HLA-selected, or crossmatched platelets.[112] The use of leukocyte-reduced blood components decreases the probability of alloimmunization to leukocyte antigens, and thus, patients with chronic transfusion requirements who have a higher likelihood of developing HLA antibodies or patients who are organ transplantation candidates are considered candidates for the empiric use of these components.[103,112,114,119] A decision to use leukocyte-reduced components in an effort to prevent alloimmunization should ideally be made before the first blood transfusion.

Certain immunosuppressed, CMV-seronegative patients, such as low-birthweight newborns, allogeneic HPC transplant recipients, women who are pregnant, and small-bowel and lung transplant recipients, are susceptible to severe transfusion-transmitted CMV disease.[120,121] Although some controversy does exist,[122] clinical studies involving such patients indicate that leukocyte-reduced blood components are as effective in preventing transmission of CMV infection as are blood components obtained from CMV-seronegative donors.[123-125] However, despite the use of universal leukocyte reduction, transfusion-transmitted CMV infections may still occur.[126] Pathogen-reduced platelets produced via the amotosalen/UVA light phototherapy system are also considered a CMV risk-reduced blood component.

Transfusion of cellular blood components is associated with immunomodulation—that is, changes in host immune function. This property was once employed to prolong the survival of renal allografts, but it has been supplanted by improved immunosuppressive drug therapy. Most, but not all, prospective randomized studies have shown that the use of leukocyte-reduced blood lowers the incidence of wound infection in selected surgical patients. However, the mechanism of this effect is unclear, and the use of leukocyte-reduced blood components for this purpose is controversial.[127,128]

Contraindications and Precautions

Patients who receive leukocyte-reduced blood components are subject to the same volume-related hazards as are those who receive non-leukocyte-reduced components. Also, leukocyte reduction does not reduce the risk of TRALI. Leukocyte reduction is not indicated to prevent TA-GVHD, as cases of TA-GVHD have been reported after its use. Aside from CMV, the risks of transfusion-transmitted infections from leukocyte-reduced blood components are the same as that from non-leukocyte-reduced components. Red Blood Cells Leukocytes Reduced may contain up to 15% fewer red cells as a result of loss in the filters. Leukocyte reduction of platelet components should not significantly affect platelet counts.

Dose and Administration

Dosing of leukocyte-reduced blood components is the same as that of non-leukocyte-reduced components. Red cell or platelet units that have undergone leukocyte reduction by prestorage methods or laboratory filtration must be transfused through a standard 170- to 260-micron filter. While uncommon, administration of these components through a bedside leukocyte-reduction filter eliminates the need for the standard blood filter. Personnel who administer blood components through bedside leukocyte-reduction filters should be thoroughly familiar with the requirements for their use in order to achieve optimal leukocyte reduction, provide acceptable blood flow rates, and ensure against excessive loss of red cells.

IRRADIATION

Description of Modification

Any cellular blood component may be gamma or x-ray irradiated in an FDA-approved irradiator. For gamma irradiation, sources include cesium-137 or cobalt-60. For x-ray irradiation, stand-alone units or radiation therapy linear accelerators may be used. The minimum radiation dose is 25 Gy at the center of the radiation field and 15 Gy at any point on the component's bag.[1] Because plasma components and Cryoprecipitated AHF are considered acellular blood components (they contain very few leukocytes to begin with, and these rare cells will not survive the freeze-thaw process), there is no need to irradiate them.

Indications

Irradiation is indicated for one reason: prevention of TA-GVHD by inactivating T lymphocytes within the component. The patient groups or components listed in Table 3 are associated with risk for developing or causing TA-GVHD.[129] Irradiation of the components going to these patients or the specific components listed should be strongly considered. Of note, in the United States, pathogen-reduced platelets treated with the amotosalen/UVA light phototherapy system are also considered TA-GVHD risk-reduced through the damage inflicted upon the leukocyte DNA. Thus, these amotosalen/UVA platelet components do not need to be gamma or x-ray irradiated.

Contraindications and Precautions

Red cell components that are irradiated can be stored at 1 to 6 C for either 28 days or until the original outdate, whichever is earlier.[1] Irradiated red cells have been demonstrated to have increased potassium leakage and hemolysis, increased fragility, and some decrease in cell recovery after transfusion.[130-132] Thus, patients who are sensitive to potassium or free hemoglobin should have their red cell components irradiated as close to the time of issue as possible (eg, low-birthweight infants). Platelet components can be irradiated at any time during their 5-day storage period, and the outdate of an irradiated platelet component is unchanged. Platelets are not damaged by irradiation at the doses used to prevent TA-GVHD.[132]

Table 3. Clinical Indications for Irradiated Components

Widely accepted indications

    Intrauterine transfusions

    Prematurity, low birthweight, or erythroblastosis fetalis in newborns

    Congenital immunodeficiencies (eg, SCID, DiGeorge syndrome)

    Hematologic malignancies or solid tumors (neuroblastoma, sarcoma, Hodgkin lymphoma)

    HPC/stem cell/marrow transplantation candidates/recipients donors

    Components that are HLA-matched or from directed donors (family members or other related donors)

    Recipients of purine analogues (eg, fludarabine)

    Granulocyte components

    Neonatal exchange transfusions

    Antithymocyte globulin

    Small-bowel transplant recipients

Potential indications

    Other malignancies, including those treated with cytotoxic agents

    Donor-recipient pairs from genetically homogeneous populations

Usually not indicated

    Patients with HIV/AIDS

    Full-term infants

    Nonimmunosuppressed patients

SCID = severe combined immunodeficiency; HPC = hematopoietic progenitor cell; HIV = human immunodeficiency virus; AIDS = acquired immunodeficiency syndrome.

Dose and Administration

The dose and administration methods of irradiated cellular blood components are the same as those of their nonirradiated counterparts.

WASHING

Description of Modification

Cellular blood components may be washed with 1 to 2 L of sterile normal saline by use of specially designed machines. The washed cells are suspended in sterile saline. For red cell components, the final product usually has a hematocrit of 70% to 80% and a volume of approximately 180 mL.[1] Saline washing removes all but traces of plasma, reduces the concentration of leukocytes, and removes platelets and cellular debris.

Indications

The predominant indication for washed cellular components in adults is to prevent recurrent or severe allergic reactions caused by plasma proteins. In IgA-deficient or haptoglobin-deficient patients at risk for anaphylaxis, washed cellular components can prevent life-threatening allergic reactions. Washed red cell components may also be considered for the prevention of transfusion-associated hyperkalemia in high-risk patients. Washed cellular components of maternal origin can also be used in fetuses or neonates who have antibody-mediated thrombocytopenias or hemolytic anemias directed against paternal antigens.

Contraindications and Precautions

Because of the risk of bacterial contamination, washed red cell components may be stored at 1 to 6 C for no longer than 24 hours after preparation, and washed platelets expire within 4 hours of washing. Thus, washed blood components should be issued as soon as possible.[1] Washing is associated with the loss of 20% of red cells and 33% of platelets.[133] For RBC units, washing has been shown to increase cell fragility and free hemoglobin in the final product,[131] which may be an issue for patients with hemolytic disease or systemic or pulmonary hypertension. Additionally, platelets have been shown to become activated during the washing process. Washed components do not have a reduced risk of viral disease transmission.[134] Washing is not an acceptable method of leukocyte reduction. Because washed components contain sufficient numbers of viable leukocytes, this process will not prevent TA-GVHD.

Dose and Administration

All units must be infused through a blood administration set containing a 170- to 260-micron filter. Because a washed RBC or platelet unit provides a lower number of red cells or platelets, respectively, patients who receive chronic transfusion of washed components may require additional transfusions.

FREEZING AND DEGLYCEROLIZATON

Description of Modification

Frozen red cells are prepared by adding glycerol, a cryoprotective agent, to RBC units that are usually less than 6 days old; however, RBC units may be rejuvenated and then frozen up to 3 days after expiration. The unit is frozen at –65 or –200 C, depending on the concentration of glycerol used, for as long as 10 years.[1] Once thawed, the unit is washed to remove the glycerol by use of a series of increasingly hypotonic saline solutions to minimize hemolysis. The unit is then reconstituted in sterile saline, usually at a hematocrit of 70% to 80%. The final product must contain at least 80% of the original red cell volume.[1] Once a unit is ordered, the thawing and deglycerolization process results in a delay before it is available. When prepared in an open system, this component may be stored at 1 to 6 C for no longer than 24 hours.[1] When prepared in a closed system, the unit may be stored at 1 to 6 C for up to 14 days.

Indications

This technique is useful for long-term preservation of RBC units of a rare phenotype, as well as autologous RBC units. Because the process of deglycerolization requires extensive washing, this component can be used for patients with a history of severe allergic reactions, including patients with IgA deficiency. For leukocyte reduction alone, the use of deglycerolized red cells is not indicated.

Contraindications and Precautions

Red cells that have been frozen and deglycerolized carry the same risks and hazards as do washed red cells. This component is capable of transmitting infectious diseases and has been shown to contain viable lymphocytes.[134,135]

Dose and Administration

All units must be administered through a blood administration set with a 170- to 260-micron filter. Deglycerolized RBC units provide a smaller red cell mass because of the loss of red cells during processing. Therefore, recipients of these units could require additional transfusions to achieve a desired hematocrit.

Oxygen Therapeutics

Oxygen therapeutics (red cell substitutes) are not FDA cleared at this time. However, in some parts of the world, these compounds can be used in human patients. Examples of two in US trials (www.clinicaltrials.gov) are bovine pegylated carboxyhemoglobin and crosslinked polymerized bovine hemoglobin, and another example, hemoglobin glutamer-250 (bovine), is used in South Africa.[136,137] Compassionate use of or expanded access to these agents may be possible and can be obtained by contacting the manufacturer to determine availability, contacting the FDA to obtain an emergency investigational new drug approval, and obtaining institutional review board approval from the institution where the patient is located.

Pathogen Inactivation

Description

Although various platforms of pathogen inactivation are currently available in Europe, the only pathogen inactivation technologies currently approved for use in the United States are solvent/detergent treatment and the amotosalen plus UVA light phototherapy system.

FDA licensing for solvent/detergent treatment includes the manufacturing of plasma derivatives and, more recently, pooled plasma for use in patients with coagulation disorders and for therapeutic plasma exchange in patients with TTP (see mentions of Octaplas in the Plasma Components section). This technology inactivates enveloped viruses, such as human immunodeficiency virus, hepatitis B virus, hepatitis C virus, and West Nile virus, by disrupting their lipid envelopes. Each lot of this plasma product comes from the pooled plasma of 630 to 1520 US source plasma donors and is dispensed in 200-mL frozen aliquots. Octaplas is comparable to other plasma components except for concentrations of protein S and $alpha_2$-plasmin inhibitor; however, each lot of Octaplas is quality controlled to have ≥ 0.4 IU/mL activity. Octaplas is sterile-filtered and frozen, which reduces the risk of bacterial and parasitic infections.[78]

The amotosalen/UVA light phototherapy system, currently approved for plasma and platelet treatment, employs psoralen-based killing of organisms containing DNA and RNA. In brief, amotosalen is a synthetic psoralen, which is a photoactive drug that intercalates into nucleic acids. Upon exposure to UVA light, amotosalen forms covalent crosslinking to pyrimidines that prevents nucleic acid replication. This results in the reduction of bacterial, viral, and parasitic pathogens, with the notable exception of prions.

Indications

The risk of transmission of various pathogens via blood transfusion continues to decrease as a result of improvements in donor screening and laboratory testing. Concern remains over the transmission of viruses in the "window period" of infection, the transmission of organisms for which routine testing is not available, and the transmission of an infectious agent before it has been identified. Because of these limitations, efforts have focused on developing technologies that treat blood components to eliminate contaminating pathogens without the need to specifically test for their presence.

Octaplas is currently FDA approved for patients with acquired multiple factor coagulopathies. It is also approved for use in therapeutic plasma exchange procedures in patients with TTP because the processing removes significant quantities of unusually large von Willebrand factor. For the latter indication, at least two reports have documented reduction or elimination of allergic transfusion reactions with the use of Octaplas during therapeutic plasma exchange.[138,139]

Pathogen-reduced plasma and platelets produced by the amotosalen/UVA light phototherapy system can be used interchangeably with other plasma or platelet components. Pathogen-reduced platelets are also TA-GVHD risk reduced, meaning that they do not require further irradiation.

Contraindications and Precautions

Octaplas is contraindicated in patients with severe protein S deficiency, IgA deficiency, or history of hypersensitivity reactions to plasma and/or Octaplas. It is important to note that nonenveloped viruses and prions are not affected by the solvent/detergent treatment.

Plasma and platelets produced by the amotosalen/UVA light phototherapy system are contraindicated in 1) neonates receiving phototherapy for hyperbilirubinemia using instruments emitting either a peak wavelength <425 nm or a bandwidth with a lower limit <375 nm, because of the risk of erythema associated with transfused amotosalen, and 2) any patient with a history of psoralen hypersensitivity.

Dose and Administration

Pathogen-reduced plasma and platelets can be transfused as routine plasma and platelet components. However, the volume of each Octaplas unit is 200 mL (typically lower than other plasma components), and platelet CCIs have been found to be lower in recipients of pathogen-reduced platelets; thus, more units of pathogen-reduced plasma or platelets may be required for transfusion.

References

1. Ooley PW, ed. Standards for blood banks and transfusion services. 30th ed. Bethesda, MD: AABB, 2016.
2. Moore GL, Ledford ME, Peck CC. The in vitro evaluation of modifications in CPD-adenine anticoagulated-preserved blood at various hematocrits. Transfusion 1980;20:419-26.
3. Neal MD, Marsh A, Marino R, et al. Massive transfusion: An evidence-based review of recent developments. Arch Surg 2012;147:563-71.
4. Mou SS, Giroir BP, Molitor-Kirsch EA, et al. Fresh whole blood versus reconstituted blood for pump priming in heart surgery in infants. N Engl J Med 2004;351:1635-44.
5. Perkins JG, Cap AP, Spinella PC, et al for the Combat Support Hospital Research Group. Comparison of platelet transfusion as fresh whole blood versus apheresis platelets

for massively transfused combat trauma patients (CME). Transfusion 2011;51:242-52.
6. Hakre S, Peel SA, O'Connell RJ, et al. Transfusion-transmissible viral infections among US military recipients of whole blood and platelets during Operation Enduring Freedom and Operation Iraqi Freedom. Transfusion 2011; 51:473-85.
7. Cubano MA, Lenhart MK, Banks DE, eds. Emergency war surgery. 4th ed. Washington, DC: US Government Printing Office, 2013.
8. McDaniel LM, Etchill EW, Raval JS, Neal MD. State of the art: Massive transfusion. Transfus Med 2014;24:138-44.
9. Leitner GC, Rach I, Horvath M, et al. Collection and storage of leukocyte depleted whole blood in autologous blood predeposit in elective surgery programs. Int J Surg 2006; 4:179-83.
10. Raval JS, Waters JH, Yazer MH. The impact of suctioning RBCs from a simulated operative site on mechanical fragility and hemolysis. Korean J Hematol 2011;46:31-5.
11. Seheult JN, Triulzi DJ, Alarcon LH, et al. Measurement of haemolysis markers following transfusion of uncrossmatched, low-titre, group O+ whole blood in civilian trauma patients: Initial experience at a level 1 trauma centre. Transfus Med 2017;27:30-5.
12. Wagner SJ. Whole blood and apheresis collections for blood components intended for transfusion. In: Fung MK, Eder AF, Spitalnik SL, Westhoff CM, eds. Technical manual. 19th ed. Bethesda, MD: AABB, 2017;6:125-60.
13. Heaton A, Miripol J, Aster R, et al. Use of Adsol preservation solution for prolonged storage of low viscosity AS-1 red blood cells. Br J Haematol 1984;57:467-78.
14. Simon TL, Marcus CS, Myhre BA, Nelson EJ. Effects of AS-3 nutrient-additive solution on 42 and 49 days of storage of red cells. Transfusion 1987;27:178-82.
15. Klein HG, Spahn DR, Carson JL. Red blood cell transfusion in clinical practice. Lancet 2007;370:415-26.

16. Carson JL, Grossman BJ, Kleinman S, et al for the Clinical Transfusion Medicine Committee. Red blood cell transfusion: A clinical practice guideline from the AABB. Ann Intern Med 2012;157:49-58.
17. Carson JL, Guyatt G, Heddle NM, et al. Clinical practice guidelines from the AABB: Red blood cell transfusion thresholds and storage. JAMA 2016;316:2025-35.
18. Daly A, Raval JS, Waters JH, et al. Effect of blood bank storage on the rheological properties of male and female donor red blood cells. Clin Hemorheol Microcirc 2014; 56:337-45.
19. Raval JS, Fontes J, Banerjee U, et al. Ascorbic acid improves membrane fragility and decreases haemolysis during red blood cell storage. Transfus Med 2013;23:87-93.
20. Raval JS, Waters JH, Seltsam A, et al. The use of the mechanical fragility test in evaluating sublethal RBC injury during storage. Vox Sang 2010;99:325-31.
21. Donadee C, Raat NJ, Kanias T, et al. Nitric oxide scavenging by red blood cell microparticles and cell-free hemoglobin as a mechanism for the red cell storage lesion. Circulation 2011;124:465-76.
22. Triulzi DJ, Yazer MH. Clinical studies of the effect of blood storage on patient outcomes. Transfus Apher Sci 2010;43:95-106.
23. Neal MD, Raval JS, Triulzi DJ, Simmons RL. Innate immune activation after transfusion of stored red blood cells. Transfus Med Rev 2013;27:113-18.
24. Steiner ME, Ness PM, Assmann SF, et al. Effects of red-cell storage duration on patients undergoing cardiac surgery. N Engl J Med 2015;372:1419-29.
25. Lacroix J, Hébert PC, Fergusson DA, et al. Age of transfused blood in critically ill adults. N Engl J Med 2015;372: 1410-18.
26. Schiffer CA, Lee EJ, Ness PM, Reilly J. Clinical evaluation of platelet concentrates stored for one to five days. Blood 1986;67:1591-4.

27. Tobian AA, Fuller AK, Uglik K, et al. The impact of platelet additive solution apheresis platelets on allergic transfusion reactions and corrected count increment. Transfusion 2014;54:1523-9.
28. Butler C, Doree C, Estcourt LJ, et al. Pathogen-reduced platelets for the prevention of bleeding. Cochrane Database Syst Rev 2013;(3):CD009072.
29. Consensus conference. Platelet transfusion therapy. JAMA 1987;257:1777-80.
30. Fresh-Frozen Plasma, Cryoprecipitate, and Platelets Administration Practice Guidelines Development Task Force of the College of American Pathologists. Practice parameter for the use of fresh-frozen plasma, cryoprecipitate, and platelets. JAMA 1994;271:777-81.
31. British Committee for Standards in Haematology BTTF. Guidelines for the use of platelet transfusions. Br J Haematol 2003;122:10-23.
32. Gmur J, Burger J, Schanz U, et al. Safety of stringent prophylactic platelet transfusion policy for patients with acute leukemia. Lancet 1991;338:1223-6.
33. Rebulla P, Finazzi G, Marangoni F, et al. The threshold for prophylactic platelet transfusions in adults with acute myeloid leukemia. Gruppo Italiano Malattie Ematologiche Maligne dell'Adulto. N Engl J Med 1997;337:1870-5.
34. Heckman KD, Weiner GJ, Davis CS, et al. Randomized study of prophylactic platelet transfusion threshold during induction therapy for adult acute leukemia: 10,000/µL versus 20,000/µL. J Clin Oncol 1997;15:1143-9.
35. Dente CJ, Shaz BH, Nicholas JM, et al. Improvements in early mortality and coagulopathy are sustained better in patients with blunt trauma after institution of a massive transfusion protocol in a civilian level I trauma center. J Trauma 2009;66:1616-24.
36. Johansson PI, Stensballe J. Hemostatic resuscitation for massive bleeding: The paradigm of plasma and platelets—a review of the current literature. Transfusion 2010;50:701-10.

37. Djulbegovic B, Gernsheimer T, Kleinman S, et al. Platelet transfusion: A clinical practice guideline from the AABB. Ann Intern Med 2015;162:205-13.
38. Warkentin TE, Greinacher A, Koster A, Lincoff AM. Treatment and prevention of heparin-induced thrombocytopenia: American College of Chest Physicians Evidence-Based Clinical Practice Guidelines (8th Edition). Chest 2008;133:340S-80S.
39. Raval JS, Mazepa MA, Russell SL, et al. Passive reporting greatly underestimates the rate of transfusion-associated circulatory overload after platelet transfusion. Vox Sang 2015;108:387-92.
40. Brecher ME, Jacobs MR, Katz LM, et al. Survey of methods used to detect bacterial contamination of platelet products in the United States in 2011. Transfusion 2013;53: 911-18.
41. Pietersz RN, Engelfriet CP, Reesink HW, et al. Detection of bacterial contamination of platelet concentrates. Vox Sang 2007;93:260-77.
42. Eder AF, Kennedy JM, Dy BA, et al. Bacterial screening of apheresis platelets and the residual risk of septic transfusion reactions: The American Red Cross experience (2004-2006). Transfusion 2007;47:1134-42.
43. Fuller AK, Uglik KM, Savage WJ, et al. Bacterial culture reduces but does not eliminate the risk of septic transfusion reactions to single-donor platelets. Transfusion 2009;49: 2588-93.
44. Harm SK, Delaney M, Charapata M, et al. Routine use of a rapid test to detect bacteria at the time of issue for nonleukoreduced, whole blood-derived platelets. Transfusion 2013;53:843-50.
45. Benjamin RJ, Kline L, Dy BA, et al. Bacterial contamination of whole-blood-derived platelets: The introduction of sample diversion and prestorage pooling with culture testing in the American Red Cross. Transfusion 2008;48:2348-55.

46. Benjamin RJ, Dy B, Perez J, et al. Bacterial culture of apheresis platelets: A mathematical model of the residual rate of contamination based on unconfirmed positive results. Vox Sang 2014;106:23-30.
47. Cid J, Lozano M. Risk of Rh(D) alloimmunization after transfusion of platelets from D+ donors to D- recipients (letter). Transfusion 2005;45:453-4.
48. Pierce RN, Reich LM, Mayer K. Hemolysis following platelet transfusions from ABO-incompatible donors. Transfusion 1985;25:60-2.
49. Herman JH, King KE. Apheresis platelet transfusions: Does ABO matter? Transfusion 2004;44:802-4.
50. Quillen K, Sheldon SL, Daniel-Johnson JA, et al. A practical strategy to reduce the risk of passive hemolysis by screening plateletpheresis donors for high-titer ABO antibodies. Transfusion 2011;51:92-6.
51. Cooling L. ABO and platelet transfusion therapy. Immunohematology 2007;23:20-33.
52. Cid J, Harm SK, Yazer MH. Platelet transfusion – the art and science of compromise. Transfus Med Hemother 2013;40:160-71.
53. Slichter SJ, Kaufman RM, Assmann SF, et al. Dose of prophylactic platelet transfusions and prevention of hemorrhage. N Engl J Med 2010;362:600-13.
54. Yankee RA, Grumet FC, Rogentine GN. Platelet transfusion: The selection of compatible platelet donors for refractory patients by lymphocyte HL-A typing. N Engl J Med 1969;281:1208-12.
55. Bishop JF, McGrath K, Wolf MM, et al. Clinical factors influencing the efficacy of pooled platelet transfusions. Blood 1988;71:383-7.
56. Kickler TS, Braine HG, Ness PM, et al. A radiolabeled antiglobulin test for crossmatching platelet transfusions. Blood 1983;61:238-42.
57. Daly PA, Schiffer CA, Aisner J, Wiernik PH. Platelet transfusion therapy. One-hour posttransfusion increments

are valuable in predicting the need for HLA-matched preparations. JAMA 1980;243:435-8.
58. Vassallo RR. Recognition and management of antibodies to human platelet antigens in platelet transfusion-refractory patients. Immunohematology 2009;25:119-24.
59. Strauss RG, Rohret PA, Randels MJ, Winegarden DC. Granulocyte collection. J Clin Apher 1991;6:241-3.
60. Dale DC, Liles WC, Llewellyn C, et al. Neutrophil transfusions: Kinetics and functions of neutrophils mobilized with granulocyte-colony-stimulating factor and dexamethasone. Transfusion 1998;38:713-21.
61. Jendiroba DB, Lichtiger B, Anaissie E, et al. Evaluation and comparison of three mobilization methods for the collection of granulocytes. Transfusion 1998;38:722-8.
62. Stroncek DF, Clay ME, Petzoldt ML, et al. Treatment of normal individuals with granulocyte-colony-stimulating factor: Donor experiences and the effects on peripheral blood CD34+ cell counts and on the collection of peripheral blood stem cells. Transfusion 1996;36:601-10.
63. Quillen K, Byrne P, Yau YY, Leitman SF. Ten-year follow-up of unrelated volunteer granulocyte donors who have received multiple cycles of granulocyte-colony-stimulating factor and dexamethasone. Transfusion 2009; 49:513-18.
64. Adkins D, Spitzer G, Johnston M, et al. Transfusions of granulocyte-colony-stimulating factor-mobilized granulocyte components to allogeneic transplant recipients: Analysis of kinetics and factors determining posttransfusion neutrophil and platelet counts. Transfusion 1997;37:737-48.
65. Lane TA. Granulocyte storage. Transfus Med Rev 1990;4: 23-34.
66. Lightfoot T, Leitman SF, Stroncek DF. Storage of G-CSF-mobilized granulocyte concentrates. Transfusion 2000;40: 1104-10.
67. Cairo MS. The use of granulocyte transfusion in neonatal sepsis. Transfus Med Rev 1990;4:14-22.

68. Oak NR, Triulzi DJ. Granulocyte transfusion therapy in abdominal organ transplant recipients. J Clin Apher 2009; 24:186-9.
69. Strauss RG, Connett JE, Gale RP, et al. A controlled trial of prophylactic granulocyte transfusions during initial induction chemotherapy for acute myelogenous leukemia. N Engl J Med 1981;305:597-603.
70. Strauss RG. Neutrophil (granulocyte) transfusions in the new millennium. Transfusion 1998;38:710-12.
71. Dale DC, Price TH. Granulocyte transfusion therapy: A new era? Curr Opin Hematol 2009;16:1-2.
72. Vamvakas EC, Pineda AA. Meta-analysis of clinical studies of the efficacy of granulocyte transfusions in the treatment of bacterial sepsis. J Clin Apher 1996;11:1-9.
73. Price TH, Boeckh M, Harrison RW, et al. Efficacy of transfusion with granulocytes from G-CSF/dexamethasone-treated donors in neutropenic patients with infection. Blood 2015;126:2153-61.
74. Price TH. Granulocyte transfusion: Current status. Semin Hematol 2007;44:15-23.
75. Heim KF, Fleisher TA, Stroncek DF, et al. The relationship between alloimmunization and posttransfusion granulocyte survival: Experience in a chronic granulomatous disease cohort. Transfusion 2011;51:1154-62.
76. Eder AF, Sebok MA. Plasma components: FFP, PF24, and thawed plasma. Immunohematology 2007;23:150-7.
77. Scott E, Puca K, Heraly J, et al. Evaluation and comparison of coagulation factor activity in fresh-frozen plasma and 24-hour plasma at thaw and after 120 hours of 1 to 6 degrees C storage. Transfusion 2009;49:1584-91.
78. Downes KA, Wilson E, Yomtovian R, Sarode R. Serial measurement of clotting factors in thawed plasma stored for 5 days. Transfusion 2001;41:570.
79. Yazer MH, Cortese-Hassett A, Triulzi DJ. Coagulation factor levels in plasma frozen within 24 hours of phlebotomy over 5 days of storage at 1 to 6 degrees C. Transfusion 2008;48:2525-30.

80. Hellstern P. Solvent/detergent-treated plasma: Composition, efficacy, and safety. Curr Opin Hematol 2004;11:346-50.
81. Consensus conference. Fresh-frozen plasma. Indications and risks. JAMA 1985;253:551-3.
82. O'Shaughnessy DF, Atterbury C, Bolton Maggs P, et al for the British Committee for Standards in Haematology Blood Transfusion Task Force. Guidelines for the use of fresh-frozen plasma, cryoprecipitate and cryosupernatant. Br J Haematol 2004;126:11-28.
83. American Society of Anesthesiologists Task Force on Perioperative Blood Transfusion, Adjuvant Therapies. Practice guidelines for perioperative blood transfusion and adjuvant therapies: An updated report. Anesthesiology 2006; 105:198-208.
84. Holland L, Sarode R. Should plasma be transfused prophylactically before invasive procedures? Curr Opin Hematol 2006;13:447-51.
85. Raval JS, Waters JH, Triulzi DJ, Yazer MH. Complications following an unnecessary perioperative plasma transfusion and literature review. Korean J Hematol 2012;47:298-301.
86. Rock G, Shumak KH, Sutton DM, et al. Cryosupernatant as replacement fluid for plasma exchange in thrombotic thrombocytopenic purpura. Members of the Canadian Apheresis Group. Br J Haematol 1996;94:383-6.
87. Patriquin CJ, Clark WF, Pavenski K, et al. How we treat thrombotic thrombocytopenic purpura: Results of a Canadian TTP practice survey. J Clin Apher 2017;32:246-56.
88. Bowden R, Sayers M. The risk of transmitting cytomegalovirus infection by fresh frozen plasma. Transfusion 1990; 30:762-3.
89. Braunstein AH, Oberman HA. Transfusion of plasma components. Transfusion 1984;24:281-6.
90. Food and Drug Administration. Fatalities reported to FDA following blood collection and transfusion: Annual summary for fiscal year 2015. Silver Spring, MD: CBER Office

of Communications, Outreach, and Development, 2016. [Available at https://www.fda.gov/downloads/Biologics BloodVaccines/SafetyAvailability/ReportaProblem/TransfusionDonationFatalities/UCM518148.pdf (accessed July 27, 2017).]

91. Eder AF, Herron RM Jr, Strupp A, et al. Effective reduction of transfusion-related acute lung injury risk with male-predominant plasma strategy in the American Red Cross (2006-2008). Transfusion 2010;50:1732-42.
92. Narick C, Triulzi DJ, Yazer MH. Transfusion-associated circulatory overload after plasma transfusion. Transfusion 2012;52:160-5.
93. Sorensen B, Bevan D. A critical evaluation of cryoprecipitate for replacement of fibrinogen. Br J Haematol 2010; 149:834-43.
94. Janson PA, Jubelirer SJ, Weinstein MJ, Deykin D. Treatment of the bleeding tendency in uremia with cryoprecipitate. N Engl J Med 1980;303:1318-22.
95. Remuzzi G. Bleeding in renal failure. Lancet 1988;i:1205-8.
96. Gibble JW, Ness PM. Fibrin glue: The perfect operative sealant? Transfusion 1990;30:741-7.
97. Meryman HT, Hornblower M. The preparation of red cells depleted of leukocytes. Review and evaluation. Transfusion 1986;26:101-6.
98. Sirchia G, Rebulla P, Parravicini A, et al. Leukocyte depletion of red cell units at the bedside by transfusion through a new filter. Transfusion 1987;27:402-5.
99. Menitove JE, McElligott MC, Aster RH. Febrile transfusion reaction: What blood component should be given next? Vox Sang 1982;42:318-21.
100. Sniecinski I, O'Donnell MR, Nowicki B, Hill LR. Prevention of refractoriness and HLA-alloimmunization using filtered blood products. Blood 1988;71:1402-7.
101. Andreu G, Dewailly J, Leberre C, et al. Prevention of HLA immunization with leukocyte-poor packed red cells and platelet concentrates obtained by filtration. Blood 1988;72:964-9.

102. Pietersz RN, Steneker I, Reesink HW. Prestorage leukocyte depletion of blood products in a closed system. Transfus Med Rev 1993;7:17-24.
103. Lane TA, Anderson KC, Goodnough LT, et al. Leukocyte reduction in blood component therapy. Ann Intern Med 1992;117:151-62.
104. Stack G, Snyder EL. Cytokine generation in stored platelet concentrates. Transfusion 1994;34:20-5.
105. Stack G, Baril L, Napychank P, Snyder EL. Cytokine generation in stored, white cell-reduced, and bacterially contaminated units of red cells. Transfusion 1995;35:199-203.
106. Yazer MH, Podlosky L, Clarke G, Nahirniak SM. The effect of prestorage WBC reduction on the rates of febrile nonhemolytic transfusion reactions to platelet concentrates and RBC. Transfusion 2004;44:10-15.
107. Paglino JC, Pomper GJ, Fisch GS, et al. Reduction of febrile but not allergic reactions to RBCs and platelets after conversion to universal prestorage leukoreduction. Transfusion 2004;44:16-24.
108. King KE, Shirey RS, Thoman SK, et al. Universal leukoreduction decreases the incidence of febrile nonhemolytic transfusion reactions to RBCs. Transfusion 2004;44:25-9.
109. Bertholf MF, Mintz PD. Comparison of plateletpheresis using two cell separators and identical donors. Transfusion 1989;29:521-3.
110. Anderson KC, Gorgone BC, Wahlers E, et al. Preparation and utilization of leukocyte-poor apheresis platelets. Transfus Sci 1991;12:163-70.
111. Rebulla P, Porretti L, Bertolini F, et al. White cell-reduced red cells prepared by filtration: A critical evaluation of current filters and methods for counting residual white cells. Transfusion 1993;33:128-33.
112. Slichter SJ. Platelet transfusion therapy. Hematol Oncol Clin North Am 1990;4:291-311.
113. Claas FH, Smeenk RJ, Schmidt R, et al. Alloimmunization against the MHC antigens after platelet transfusions is due

to contaminating leukocytes in the platelet suspension. Exp Hematol 1981;9:84-9.
114. Seftel MD, Growe GH, Petraszko T, et al. Universal prestorage leukoreduction in Canada decreases platelet alloimmunization and refractoriness. Blood 2004;103:333-9.
115. Perkins HA, Payne R, Ferguson J, Wood M. Nonhemolytic febrile transfusion reactions. Quantitative effects of blood components with emphasis on isoantigenic incompatibility of leukocytes. Vox Sang 1966;11:578-600.
116. Muylle L, Joos M, Wouters E, et al. Increased tumor necrosis factor alpha (TNF alpha), interleukin 1, and interleukin 6 (IL-6) levels in the plasma of stored platelet concentrates: Relationship between TNF alpha and IL-6 levels and febrile transfusion reactions. Transfusion 1993;33:195-9.
117. Heddle NM, Blajchman MA. The leukodepletion of cellular blood products in the prevention of HLA-alloimmunization and refractoriness to allogeneic platelet transfusions. Blood 1995;85:603-6.
118. Heddle NM, Klama L, Singer J, et al. The role of the plasma from platelet concentrates in transfusion reactions. N Engl J Med 1994;331:625-8.
119. Leukocyte reduction and ultraviolet B irradiation of platelets to prevent alloimmunization and refractoriness to platelet transfusions. The Trial to Reduce Alloimmunization to Platelets Study Group. N Engl J Med 1997;337:1861-9.
120. Sayers MH, Anderson KC, Goodnough LT, et al. Reducing the risk for transfusion-transmitted cytomegalovirus infection. Ann Intern Med 1992;116:55-62.
121. Ziemann M, Unmack A, Steppat D, et al. The natural course of primary cytomegalovirus infection in blood donors. Vox Sang 2010;99:24-33.
122. Nichols WG, Price TH, Gooley T, et al. Transfusion-transmitted cytomegalovirus infection after receipt of leukoreduced blood products. Blood 2003;101:4195-200.
123. Bowden RA, Slichter SJ, Sayers M, et al. A comparison of filtered leukocyte-reduced and cytomegalovirus (CMV) seronegative blood products for the prevention of transfu-

sion-associated CMV infection after marrow transplant. Blood 1995;86:3598-603.
124. Narvios AB, Przepiorka D, Tarrand J, et al. Transfusion support using filtered unscreened blood products for cytomegalovirus-negative allogeneic marrow transplant recipients. Bone Marrow Transplant 1998;22:575-7.
125. Laupacis A, Brown J, Costello B, et al. Prevention of posttransfusion CMV in the era of universal WBC reduction: A consensus statement. Transfusion 2001;41:560-9.
126. Wu Y, Zou S, Cable R, et al. Direct assessment of cytomegalovirus transfusion-transmitted risks after universal leukoreduction. Transfusion 2010;50:776-86.
127. Blajchman MA. Allogeneic blood transfusions, immunomodulation, and postoperative bacterial infection: Do we have the answers yet? Transfusion 1997;37:121-5.
128. Blajchman MA, Dzik S, Vamvakas EC, et al. Clinical and molecular basis of transfusion-induced immunomodulation: Summary of the proceedings of a state-of-the-art conference. Transfus Med Rev 2001;15:108-35.
129. Treleaven J, Gennery A, Marsh J, et al. Guidelines on the use of irradiated blood components prepared by the British Committee for Standards in Haematology Blood Transfusion Task Force. Br J Haematol 2011;152:35-51.
130. Arseniev L, Schumann G, Andres J. Kinetics of extracellular potassium concentration in irradiated red blood cells. Infusionsther Transfusionsmed 1994;21:322-4.
131. Harm SK, Raval JS, Cramer J, et al. Haemolysis and sublethal injury of RBCs after routine blood bank manipulations. Transfus Med 2012;22:181-5.
132. Guidelines on gamma irradiation of blood components for the prevention of transfusion-associated graft-versus-host disease. British Committee for Standards in Haematology Blood Transfusion Task Force. Transfus Med 1996;6:261-71.
133. Harm SK, Dunbar NM. Transfusion-service-related activities: Pretransfusion testing and storage, monitoring, processing, distribution, and inventory management of blood components. In: Fung MK, Eder AF, Spitalnik SL, West-

hoff CM, eds. Technical manual. 19th ed. Bethesda, MD: AABB, 2017;17:457-88.
134. Haugen RK. Hepatitis after the transfusion of frozen red cells and washed red cells. N Engl J Med 1979;301:393-5.
135. Chaplin H Jr. Frozen red cells revisited. N Engl J Med 1984;311:1696-8.
136. A phase 1 safety study of SANGUINATE in patients with acute severe anemia. ClinicalTrials.gov identifier NCT02754999. Bethesda, MD: US National Institutes of Health, 2017. [Available at https://clinicaltrials.gov/ct2/show/NCT02754999 (accessed July 24, 2017).]
137. Mer M, Hodgson E, Wallis L, et al. Hemoglobin glutamer-250 (bovine) in South Africa: Consensus usage guidelines from clinician experts who have treated patients. Transfusion 2016;56:2631-6.
138. Scully M, Longair I, Flynn M, et al. Cryosupernatant and solvent detergent fresh-frozen plasma (Octaplas) usage at a single centre in acute thrombotic thrombocytopenic purpura. Vox Sang 2007;93:154-8.
139. Sidhu D, Snyder EL, Tormey CA. Two approaches to the clinical dilemma of treating TTP with therapeutic plasma exchange in patients with a history of anaphylactic reactions to plasma. J Clin Apher 2017;32:158-62.

PLASMA DERIVATIVES

Plasma derivatives are stocked in either the blood bank or the pharmacy, depending on institutional preference. The available products constantly change, reflecting the regulatory approval of new products in each country and evidence of efficacy available from clinical trials. Most hospitals carry a limited supply of the most commonly used derivatives [eg, immune globulins, Factor VIII and IX products, and prothrombin complex concentrates (PCCs)] and order other products from blood suppliers on demand. Community hospitals may not routinely stock any derivatives. Derivative suppliers can usually deliver the products within 24 hours of the request. Table 4 lists the products discussed in this chapter.

Factor VIII Concentrates

The large assortment of Factor VIII products available is described below. Product choice is determined by the treating hematologist and the patient. Older hemophilia patients may still receive some of the older types of plasma-derived factors, despite the increased pathogen risk, because they are familiar with the product, have responded predictably to that product for many years, and may be concerned that changing to a new product could lead to inhibitor development (antibodies directed against the coagulation factor). Furthermore, because many older

Table 4. Plasma Derivatives

Component/Product	Composition	Volume	Indications
Fibrinogen concentrate (human)	Fibrinogen (1 g/vial)	50 mL	Acute bleeding episodes for congenital fibrinogen deficiency
Factor VIIa (recombinant)	Factor VIIa (1 mg, 2 mg, 5 mg, 8 mg)	1 mL; 2 mL; 5 mL; 8 mL	Bleeding or prophylaxis before surgery for hemophilia A or B with inhibitors; Factor VII deficiency; Glanzmann thrombasthenia
Factor VIII (recombinant; human)	Factor VIII; trace amount of other plasma proteins (products vary in purity)	Varies	Hemophilia A (Factor VIII deficiency); von Willebrand disease (selected products only)
Factor IX (recombinant; human)	Factor IX; trace amount of other plasma proteins (products vary in purity)	Varies	Hemophilia B (Factor IX deficiency)

Factor X concentrate (human)	Factor X (250 or 500 IU)	2.5 mL; 5 mL	On-demand treatment and control of bleeding episodes in adults and children aged 12 years and above with hereditary Factor X deficiency
Factor XIII concentrate (human; recombinant)	Factor XIII	20 mL	Routine prophylaxis for congenital Factor XIII deficiency
Prothrombin complex concentrates (PCCs) (human)	4-factor PCC: Factors II, VII, IX, and X (500/1000 IU Factor IX)	20 mL; 40 mL	Urgent reversal of vitamin K antagonist anticoagulation in patients with acute major bleeding
	3-factor PCC: Factors II, IX, X, and trace amount of Factor VII (500/1500 IU Factor IX)	5-10 mL	Alternative (second choice) for hemophilia B (Factor IX deficiency)

(Continued)

Table 4. Plasma Derivatives (Continued)

Component/Product	Composition	Volume	Indications
Activated prothrombin complex concentrates (aPCCs) (human)	Factors II, IX, X (nonactivated), and Factor VII (activated)	20 mL; 50 mL	Bleeding or prophylaxis before surgery for hemophilia A or B with inhibitors
Antithrombin (human; recombinant)	Antithrombin; trace amount of other plasma proteins	10 mL	Treatment of antithrombin deficiency
Protein C concentrate	Protein C	5 mL; 10 mL	Prevention and treatment of venous thrombosis and purpura fulminans in patients with severe congenital protein C deficiency
C1 esterase inhibitors (human; recombinant)	C1 esterase inhibitor (human, 500 IU; recombinant, 2100 IU)	8 mL or 10 mL (28 mL recombinant)	Treatment or prophylaxis (product dependent) of acute attacks of hereditary angioedema

Rh Immune Globulin	IgG anti-D; preparations for IV and/or IM use (250 IU/1500 IU)	1 mL	Prevention of hemolytic disease of the fetus and newborn due to D antigen; treatment of immune thrombocytopenia (selected products only in D-positive patients)
Immune globulin	IgG antibodies; preparations for IV and/or IM use	Varies	Treatment of hypo- or agammaglobulinemia; disease prophylaxis; autoimmune thrombocytopenia (IV only)
Albumin/PPF	Albumin; some α-, β-globulins	Varies	Volume expansion

IV = intravenous; IM = intramuscular; IgG = immunoglobulin G; PPF = plasma protein fraction.

hemophilia patients were infected with human immunodeficiency virus (HIV) or hepatitis C virus in the 1980s, their level of concern about new infectious transmission may be lower than their concern about inhibitor development.

Factor VIII preparations can be derived from human plasma or produced by recombinant technology. Various procedures are used to inactivate viruses in plasma-derived Factor VIII products and reduce the risk of infectious disease transmission[1]; these procedures include a combination of nanofiltration, pasteurization and solvent/detergent treatment, and affinity chromatography preparation. It should be noted that no treatment procedure or combination of procedures eliminates the risk of virus transmission. This may be particularly relevant with respect to certain non-lipid-enveloped viruses (such as hepatitis A and parvovirus B19), as well as emerging pathogens.

Human-plasma-derived Factor VIII concentrate [also referred to as antihemophilic factor (AHF)] is prepared by fractionation of pooled human plasma that is frozen soon after collection. Several types of human-plasma-derived Factor VIII concentrates are available. All products take the form of a sterile, stable, lyophilized concentrate, but they differ in terms of protein purity. The purity is usually expressed by the specific activity, which refers to units of clotting factor per milligram of protein.

The purest human-derived products are produced through immunoaffinity chromatography that uses murine monoclonal antibodies to a portion of the Factor VIII complex.[1] The purity of these products is greater than 90% before the addition of albumin, which is used as a stabilizer.

Recombinant Factor VIII (rFVIII) is produced in established animal or human cell lines. First-generation rFVIII contains animal and/or human-plasma-derived proteins in the culture medium and in the final-formulation vial. Second-generation rFVIII contains plasma proteins in the medium but not in the final formulation. Third-generation rFVIII does not contain any plasma-derived proteins in the culture medium or in the final-formulation vial, and the fourth generation is produced in a human cell line with no animal or human-derived materials added during the manufacturing process or to the final product. Manufacturers have strived to develop a product that is most similar to human Factor VIII to avoid inhibitor development and reduce early clearance of the product.[1]

Until recently, rFVIII had become the product of choice for treating patients with hemophilia A,[1] because of its safety profile regarding transmitting human infectious organisms. However, a previous controversy has recently reemerged regarding a higher risk of inhibitor development with recombinant products. A 2013 meta-analysis reported that the use of recombinant vs plasma-derived Factor VIII products was not associated with a different risk of inhibitor development.[2] However, that conclusion has now come into question after the results were published from a recent randomized clinical trial (SIPPET study) comparing the incidence of Factor VIII inhibitors among patients treated with plasma-derived Factor VIII containing von Willebrand factor (vWF) or recombinant Factor VIII.[3] Subjects were male hemophilia A patients less than 6 years of age with no previous treatment with any Factor VIII concentrate or only minimal treatment with blood components from 42 international sites. The study concluded that early-replacement therapy with plasma-derived Factor VIII was associated with a lower incidence of inhibitor development than was therapy with rFVIII. Because inhibitor formation severely complicates hemophilia treatment, many clinicians are rethinking the approach to treating hemophilia A.

Several novel Factor VIII products designed to prolong half-life or decrease immunogenicity have recently become available.[4] The technologies to extend the factor half-life include conjugation of clotting factors to polyethylene glycol (PEG) and fusion of clotting factors to albumin or the Fc component of immunoglobulin G (IgG). A half-life range of 8 to 12 hours has been reported for all previously available Factor VIII products; however, the extending technologies may prolong the half-life by 1.4- to 1.7-fold.[4] The half-life can be only modestly prolonged because of the dependence of Factor VIII clearance on the clearance of vWF, which is not altered by using longer-acting Factor VIII. Active bleeding, surgery, or inhibitor development may reduce the half-life. Extended half-life Factor VIII products have been shown to be well tolerated and efficacious in preventing bleeding episodes in patients with hemophilia A.[5] The following products are currently available: Eloctate (rFVIII Fc fusion protein, Biogen Idec, Cambridge, MA); Adynovate (rFVIII PEGylated, Shire, Lexington, MA); and Afstyla (rFVIII single chain, CSL Behring, King of Prussia, PA). These products are generally given once or twice per week to prevent bleeding events. This dosing offers the potential to reduce injections by 50% compared to traditional Factor VIII concentrates. A new product in development offers a revolutionary approach to hemophilia A treatment. The product, emicizumab (Roche, Indianapolis, IN), is a recombinant humanized bispecific antibody that binds to activated Factor IX and Factor X and mimics the cofactor function of Factor VIII with a half-life of 4 to 5 weeks.[6] Clinical trials of this product are ongoing.

Several intermediate-purity Factor VIII concentrates produced in a manner that retains vWF are also on the market.[7] Humate-P (CSL Behring, King of Prussia, PA) and Alphanate (Grifols Biologicals, Los Angeles, CA) are labeled in vWF ristocetin cofactor activity units and are indicated for the treatment of von Willebrand disease (vWD). In addition, a vWF/Factor VIII high-purity concentrate replacement therapy developed specifically for vWD (Wilate, Octapharma, Hoboken, NJ) is available. This product has a physiologic ratio of vWF to Factor VIII of 1:1. A new recombinant vWF concentrate (VONVENDI, Baxalta, Westlake Village, CA) was recently licensed in the United States and is indicated to treat and control bleeding episodes in adults diagnosed with vWD.[8]

Recombinant porcine Factor VIII (Obizur, Shire, Bannockburn, IL) is approved for the treatment of bleeding in acquired hemophilia A based on a prospective study in adults with serious bleeding[9]; the 28 subjects all achieved hemostasis and Factor VIII levels >100% within 24 hours after receiving porcine Factor VIII. The response is based on cross-reactive Factor VIII inhibitor titer. Subjects without cross-reactivity achieved very high Factor VIII levels.

(For indications, dosing, and treatment, see Chapter 3: Hemostatic Disorders.)

Factor IX Concentrates

Factor IX preparations are available from recombinant and plasma-derived sources. Human-derived Factor IX concentrates are heat-treated and/or solvent/detergent-treated to decrease the risk of infectious diseases. The highly purified preparation also contains trace (nontherapeutic) amounts of Factors II, VII, and X. These concentrates were developed by advanced chromatographic methods or monoclonal antibody purification in order to provide a less thrombogenic material.

Recombinant Factor IX concentrate is produced in a Chinese hamster ovary cell line. Because no human products are used, it is not thought to transmit human infectious diseases. For this reason, recombinant Factor IX is the treatment of choice for new patients with hemophilia B and for those with limited exposure to human-derived Factor IX products.[1] A clinical trial comparing inhibitor development between patients receiving recombinant vs human-derived Factor IX products has not been conducted, but the risk of inhibitor development is much lower in patients with hemophilia B.

Three extended half-life recombinant Factor IX products have been approved by the Food and Drug Administration (FDA): Alprolix (Biogen Idec, Cambridge, MA) is Factor IX fused to the Fc portion of IgG; Idelvion (CSL Behring, King of Prussia, PA) is a recombinant Factor IX fused to albumin; and REBINYN (Novo Nordisk, Plainsboro, NJ) is a PEGylated Factor IX with PEG conjugated to the activated peptide of Factor IX. REBINYN had improved recovery in clinical trials because upon activation, the activation peptide and PEG are cleaved off, and the remaining Factor IX resembles and behaves similarly to endogenous Factor IX.

The half-life of traditional Factor IX concentrates has been reported to range from 18 to 24 hours.[7] This is prolonged by up to four to five times in the new longer-acting products. The extended half-life products are given every 1 to 2 weeks vs twice a week for the traditional products.[5]

Factor X Concentrate

Historically, Factor X was available only as part of PCC (see below), a product with a variable amount of Factor X. Recently, a plasma-derived Factor X concentrate (Coagadex, Bio Products Laboratory, Elstree, UK) was approved for treatment and control of bleeding episodes in patients with hereditary Factor X deficiency. Two multicenter, prospective, open-label clinical trials assessing the efficacy of Factor X concentrate have been completed, and 98% to 100% of bleeding episodes were successfully treated.[10]

Prothrombin Complex Concentrate

PCC is a term that refers to crude preparations of Factor IX that contain other vitamin K-dependent proteins to varying extents but are generally labeled by Factor IX content. Products approved in the United States include Bebulin VH (Baxter Healthcare, Deerfield, IL), Profilnine SD (Grifols Biologicals, Los Angeles, CA), and Kcentra (CSL Behring, King of Prussia, PA). The first two products are referred to as 3-factor concentrates and contain mainly Factors II, IX, and X, and low amounts of

Factor VII. Kcentra includes therapeutic levels of Factor VII in addition, and is referred to as a 4-factor concentrate. Kcentra is indicated for the urgent reversal of acquired coagulation factor deficiency induced by vitamin K antagonist (VKA, eg, warfarin) therapy in adult patients with acute major bleeding or the need for urgent surgery or other invasive procedure.[11] It contains heparin and is contraindicated in patients with heparin-induced thrombocytopenia (HIT). A review of PCCs reported the risk of thrombotic complications may be increased by underlying disease, high or frequent dosing, and poorly balanced pro- and anticoagulant constituents.[12] One exploratory analysis of two randomized, plasma-controlled trials found the risk of thromboembolic events was 7% for both subjects that received plasma and those that received PCCs.[13] Off-label use of PCCs in the reversal of direct Factor Xa inhibitors (rivaroxaban/apixiban)[14] has been reported. Nonactivated PCCs are not effective for the reversal of dabigatran.[14] Dabigitran should be reversed using idarucizumab (Praxbind, Boehringer Ingelheim Pharmaceuticals, Ridgefield, CT).[15]

(For indications, dosing, and treatment, see Chapter 3: Hemostatic Disorders.)

Other Recombinant and Plasma Protein Derivatives

Antithrombin Concentrate

Antithrombin (AT) is an important inhibitor of coagulation and inflammation. Thrombin and activated Factors IX, X, XI, and XII are inhibited by AT. The rate at which these factors are inhibited is dramatically increased in the presence of heparin. Congenital deficiencies of AT are associated with venous thrombotic disease.[16] AT concentrates are prepared from pooled units of human plasma from normal donors and are used to treat patients with hereditary AT deficiency who have thrombosis or who require prophylaxis when they are scheduled to undergo surgical or obstetric procedures. A recombinant AT product (Atryn, rEVO Biologics, Framingham, MA) is licensed in the United States for the prevention of perioperative and peripartum thromboembolic events in hereditary AT-deficient patients. The recombinant protein has a different glycosylation pattern, resulting in greater heparin affinity; however, the novel epitopes could potentially induce an immune response in recipients. The plasma half-life of the recombinant product is considerably shorter than that of the plasma-derived product (10.5 vs 60 hours).[17]

Recombinant Factor VIIa and aPCCs

Recombinant Factor VIIa (NovoSeven; NovoNordisk, Princeton, NJ) (rFVIIa) is licensed to treat or prevent bleeding episodes in patients with an inhibitor to Factor VIII or Factor IX (either acquired or with hemophilia A or B), in patients with congenital Factor VII deficiency, and in patients with Glanzmann thrombasthenia.[18] rFVIIa interacts with tissue factor, binds to surfaces of activated platelets, and directly activates Factor X. Activated Factor X complexes with Factor Va, a process that leads to a thrombin burst and clot formation. *It is important to note that the resulting shortened prothrombin time (PT) does not predict clinical effectiveness.* rFVIIa has a mean half-life of 2.7 hours. This product has been used off-label to treat patients with myriad bleeding problems, including platelet function disorders, liver disease, intracranial hemorrhage, trauma, postpartum hemorrhage, and reversal of anticoagulant agents. Anecdotal reports have demonstrated efficacy in many of these clinical situations, but many failures also occur, and the few well-controlled trials that have been conducted have generally been disappointing.[19] The most appropriate dose and schedule for treating any indication are not fully established, and this product should be used in consultation with a physician who is experienced in its use. Adverse effects include a risk of venous and arterial thromboembolic events.[20]

Activated prothrombin complex concentrates (aPCCs) (FEIBA, Baxter Healthcare, Westlake Village, CA) contain nonactivated Factors II, IX, and X, and activated Factor VII. These factors are also able to bypass an inhibitor to Factor VIII or IX to achieve hemostasis. This product is derived from heat-treated human plasma. The choice of product (rFVIIa vs aPCCs) to treat an inhibitor depends on the type and current titer of the inhibitor, the location of the bleeding, and previous response to these products.[1] (See Chapter 3: Hemostatic Disorders.)

Fibrinogen Concentrate

Fibrinogen concentrate (RiaSTAP, CSL Behring, King of Prussia, PA) is a pasteurized human product stored as a lyophilized powder at room temperature. Vials contain 900 to 1300 mg fibrinogen. Fibrinogen concentrate is approved in the United States for the treatment of acute bleeding episodes in patients with congenital fibrinogen deficiency, including afibrinogenemia and hypofibrinogenemia. Fibrinogen concentrate has been used in settings of acquired hypofibrinogenemia (eg, cardiac surgery, postpartum hemorrhage, trauma, and liver transplantation).

Protein C Concentrate

Protein C is a vitamin-K-dependent inhibitor of coagulation that is converted to its active form by the thrombin/thrombomodulin complex. Human-plasma-derived protein C concentrate (Ceprotin, Baxter Healthcare, Westlake Village, CA) is available for treatment of patients with severe congenital protein C deficiency.

Fibrin Sealant

Fibrin sealants (also called fibrin glue) consist of concentrated fibrinogen and thrombin, which on mixing create a fibrin clot. Fibrin sealant has been used in a diverse number of surgical procedures as a hemostat, sealant, and adhesive; the most extensive use has been in cardiothoracic surgery and neurosurgery.[21,22] The FDA has licensed multiple commercially prepared fibrin sealant kits that use lyophilized, virus-inactivated human fibrinogen and thrombin. A commercial kit has the benefit of standardized preparation and ease of administration, as well as a low risk of virus transmission. Some topical bovine thrombin preparations may contain bovine Factor V, which can result in the formation of antibodies that cross-react with human Factor V and lead to serious clinical sequelae.[23] Both recombinant and plasma-derived human thrombin products are also available.

Factor XIII Concentrate

A Factor XIII concentrate, Corifact (CSL Behring, King of Prussia, PA), is available in the United States and is known as Fibrogammin P in other countries. It is indicated for routine prophylactic treatment of congenital Factor XIII deficiency. In addition, Factor XIII concentrate has also been shown to improve clot stability when used in conjunction with rFVIIa in hemophilia A patients with inhibitors.[24] The half-life of plasma-derived Factor XIII is approximately 9 days, and Corifact is dosed every 28 days. A recombinant Factor XIII A-subunit, TRETTEN (Novo Nordisk, Bagsvaerd, Denmark), is approved in the United States for routine prophylaxis of bleeding in patients with congenital Factor XIII A-subunit deficiency. The standard dose is 35 IU/kg monthly. Fresh Frozen Plasma and Cryoprecipitated AHF are also sources of Factor XIII, providing 1 and 3 units/mL of Factor XIII, respectively, and can be used to successfully treat Factor XIII deficiency when factor concentrates are not available.[25]

C1 Esterase Inhibitors

Patients with hereditary angioedema (HAE) caused by inadequate or nonfunctioning C1 esterase inhibitor (C1-INH) experience acute attacks of localized swelling (angioedema) as a result of mutations in the C1-INH gene. De novo mutations account for approximately 25% of HAE cases. The lack of functional C1-INH results in uncontrolled activation of the contact system, leading to an excessive release of bradykinin that causes increased vascular permeability and angioedema. There are three treatments available: two plasma-derived C1-INH products (Cinryze, Shire, Bannockburn, IL, and Berinert, CSL Behring, King of Prussia, PA) and one recombinant C1-INH (Ruconest, Pharming Group, Leiden, Netherlands).[26]

Albumin and Plasma Protein Fraction

Albumin

Albumin is derived from human plasma and composed of 96% albumin and 4% globulin and other proteins. It is prepared by the cold alcohol fractionation process and subsequently heated to 60 C for 10 hours to prevent viral disease transmission.

Plasma Protein Fraction

Plasma protein fraction (PPF) is a similar product, except that it is subjected to fewer purification steps in the fractionation process. PPF contains about 83% albumin and 17% globulin. Normal serum albumin is available as a 25% or a 5% solution, whereas PPF is available as a 5% solution. Each of the products has a sodium content of about 145 mmol/L (145 mEq/L). The 5% albumin solution is osmotically and oncotically equivalent to plasma, and the 25% solution has osmotic and oncotic effects that are five times those of plasma. Albumin has a plasma half-life of 15 to 20 days. These products contain no coagulation factors.

Indications

Albumin is used for its oncotic activity in patients who are both hypovolemic and hypoproteinemic (eg, in clinical settings of shock, thermal injury, nephrotic syndrome, and large-volume paracentesis). It is also used as a replacement fluid in patients undergoing therapeutic plasma exchange. However, the specific clinical situations for which albumin therapy is recommended and in which it has proved to be beneficial remain a subject of controversy. A large study comparing albumin to saline for fluid resuscitation in the intensive care unit found no adverse effect of albumin and found similar outcomes with the use of albumin or normal saline for fluid resuscitation.[27] A 2013 Cochrane Review found no evidence that resuscitation with colloids reduces the risk of death, compared to resuscitation with crystalloids, in patients with trauma or burns, or following surgery.[28] Indications for the use of PPF parallel those given for 5% albumin.

Contraindications and Precautions

Albumin is not indicated for correction of hypoproteinemia or nutritional hypoalbuminemia. Use of the 25% albumin solution is contraindicated in dehydrated patients unless it is supplemented by the infusion of crystalloid solutions to provide volume expansion. The 25% albumin solution can be diluted only with normal saline or D5W; sterile water should not be used. Reported side effects include flushing, urticaria, chills, fever, and headache. PPF, but not albumin, is contraindicated for intra-arterial administration or infusion during cardiopulmonary bypass. Albumin and PPF are extremely safe regarding transmission of viruses.

Dose and Administration

Albumin and PPF need not be given through a filter. Treatment of hypotension with albumin and PPF should be guided by the patient's hemodynamic response. A 500-mL dose (10 to 20 mL/kg or 0.5 to 1 g/kg/dose in children) is given rapidly for shock. In the absence of symptomatic hypovolemia, an infusion rate of 1 to 2 mL/minute is suitable. In burn patients, the dose of albumin or PPF is the amount necessary to maintain the circulating total plasma protein level at 5.2 g/dL or higher. Albumin will not correct chronic hypoalbuminemia and should not be used for long-term therapy.

Synthetic Volume Expanders

Description

Crystalloid solutions such as normal saline and lactated Ringer's solution are isotonic with plasma. Normal saline contains only sodium and chloride ions, while lactated Ringer's solution also contains potassium, calcium, and lactate. Hypotonic solutions of sodium chloride are also available. Crystalloid solutions are less expensive than the colloid solutions.

Colloids used for volume expansion include hydroxyethyl starch (HES), gelatins, and dextran. HES is available as a 6% solution in normal saline. The intravascular half-life of HES is more than 24 hours.

Indications

By virtue of their oncotic properties, colloids are useful as volume expanders in the treatment of hemorrhagic shock and burns. Crystalloid solutions alone expand the plasma volume temporarily as they rapidly cross capillary membranes, but only one-third of the salt solution remains in the intravascular space. Accordingly, 2 to 3 volumes of crystalloid are required to replace 1 volume of lost plasma. Crystalloid and colloid solutions are relatively nontoxic and inexpensive (colloids are more expensive than crystalloids), are readily available, can be stored at room temperature, require no compatibility testing, and are free of the risk of infectious disease. The relative merits of crystalloid and colloid solutions for acute hypovolemia remain a subject of controversy, but a meta-analysis found no evidence that colloids reduced the risk of death compared to crystalloids.[28] A randomized trial in cardiac surgery patients found that neither colloid nor crystalloid improved renal oxygen consumption, but crystalloids increased the glomerular filtration rate (GFR) and were associated with impaired renal oxygenation.[29]

Contraindications and Precautions

Circulatory overload is a risk associated with all volume expanders. The side effects associated with HES occur less frequently than do those associated with dextran, but the side effects of HES do include prolongation of PT and activated partial thromboplastin time (aPTT), as well as pruritus. In 2013, the FDA issued a recommendation that HES should not be used in critically ill patients and in patients with preexisting renal dysfunction, because of the increased risk of adverse events in these populations. A multicenter retrospective review reported that hydroxyethyl starch used at low doses during therapeutic leukocyte reduction procedures was not associated with adverse events.[30] Dextran can produce anaphylactic reactions, fever, rash, tachycardia, and hypotension, as well as increased bleeding tendencies resulting from its interference with platelet function and its stimulation of fibrinolysis. Renal failure has also been reported with the infusion of low-molecular-weight dextran products. High-molecular-weight dextrans have been known to aggregate red cells in vitro, leading to interference with blood typing and crossmatching.

Administration

Crystalloid and colloid solutions do not have to be administered through a blood filter.

Immune Globulins

Description

Immune globulins are prepared by cold ethanol fractionation from pools of human plasma from 15,000 to 60,000 healthy volunteers. Gamma globulin preparations and specific hyperimmune globulin preparations with high titers against specific infectious agents or toxins are available for intramuscular (IM) use. These products have several disadvantages: IM administration requires 4 to 7 days to achieve peak plasma levels; the maximum dose that can be given is limited by muscle mass; administration may be painful; and IM immune globulin (IMIG) can undergo proteolytic breakdown at the IM site. IM products are now given primarily for disease prophylaxis. These preparations are sterile solutions with protein concentrations of approximately 16.5 g/dL. The predominant immune globulin is IgG, but IgA and IgM may also be present.

Intravenous (IV) immune globulin (IVIG) minimizes some of the disadvantages of IMIG. Sterile, lyophilized IVIG differs from IMIG in the mode of preparation, use of additives, pH, and protein content (stated on the package insert). More than 90% of the protein is IgG; there are only trace quantities of IgA and IgM. Infusion of IVIG products can achieve peak levels of IgG immediately after infusion. The gamma globulin molecules of IVIG preparations are intact. IVIG contains antibodies to a wide variety of infectious agents, but specific titers are not known for most preparations. The half-lives of IVIG and IMIG preparations vary from 18 to 32 days, which is the same range as that for native IgG.[31,32]

Indications

Immune globulin preparations can be used to provide passive antibody prophylaxis for susceptible persons who are exposed to certain diseases and as replacement therapy in primary or acquired immunodeficiency states. Immune globulin is also used to modulate the immune system in autoimmune diseases. The modes of action of IVIG are not fully understood.[33] Both FDA-approved and off-label, non-FDA-approved indications continue to expand. The efficacy of IVIG in various clinical settings has been extensively reviewed.[34-38]

Contraindications and Precautions

Adverse reactions to immune globulin preparations include headache, fatigue, chills, backache, lightheadedness, fever, flushing, and nausea. An IgA-depleted product is available and has been used safely in IgA-deficient patients with anti-IgA.[39] IM preparations must not be given intravenously because they contain immunoglobulin aggregates that may activate the complement and kinin systems. Infectious risk is effectively mitigated using virus-inactivation techniques. Hemolysis caused by the passive transfer of blood group antibodies can be a severe complication of IVIG. Renal dysfunction and acute renal failure have been reported with sucrose-containing IVIG preparations, and these products should be given with caution to patients at risk for developing acute renal failure.[40] Information about management of the infusion rate is included in the package insert; these recommendations should be stringently followed because some data suggest that rapid infusion of this hyperviscous product may increase the risk of renal damage and thrombosis.

Dose and Administration

The dose of immune globulin depends on the reason for administration, patient characteristics, and the preparation used (IM or IV).

Rh Immune Globulin

Description

Rh Immune Globulin (RhIG) is prepared from pooled human plasma and marketed under the trade names of WinRho SDF (Cangene, Winnipeg, Canada), Rhophylac (CSL Behring, King of Prussia, PA), and RhoGAM (Kedrion Biopharma, Fort Lee, NJ). RhIG contains mostly IgG anti-D. A variety of dosages are available for either IM or IV administration (WinRho and Rhophylac). RhoGAM is available in 300-μg (1500 IU) and 50-μg (150 IU) (microdose) preparations for IM injection only and is used for the prevention of alloimmunization to the RhD antigen.

Solvent/detergent-treated IV preparations are FDA approved for both suppression of immunization to the D antigen and treatment of immune thrombocytopenia (ITP). The package insert should be consulted for dosing recommendations for all products. These preparations appear to be very safe with respect to infectious disease transmission. The availability of a safe and effective monoclonal anti-D IgG, which could be produced in limitless quantities, would be very desirable. However, experiments with monoclonal anti-D for Rh prophylaxis have not been successful up to this time.

Indications and Dosage

Antepartum Prevention of Alloimmunization to the D Antigen

For D-negative females, a 50-µg microdose of RhIG can be used in the situations of abortion, miscarriage, and termination of ectopic pregnancy during the first 12 weeks of gestation (fetal red cell mass at 12 weeks of gestation is estimated to be <2.5 mL). After 12 weeks of gestation, a full dose (300-µg) of IM or IV RhIG should be administered for these indications. A full dose is also recommended for use after amniocentesis and for any other obstetric complication (eg, abdominal trauma and antepartum hemorrhage) or obstetric manipulation (eg, external version) occurring after 12 weeks of pregnancy.[41,42] RhIG should be given (preferably) within 72 hours of amniocentesis or any other obstetric event that may cause fetomaternal hemorrhage (FMH), including termination of pregnancy, unless it has been determined either that the fetus is D negative or that maternal immunization to the D antigen has already occurred. If repeated amniocenteses are performed, additional doses should be considered, particularly if the procedures are performed more than 21 days apart.

All nonimmunized D-negative females with a D-positive fetus should receive antepartum prophylaxis with a full dose of either IM or IV RhIG at 28 weeks of gestation. Together, postpartum prophylaxis and antepartum prophylaxis have reduced the number of D-negative females who become alloimmunized to the

D antigen during gestation to 0.1%; the rate with postpartum prophylaxis alone was 1% to 2%.[43] It has been suggested that integration of *RHD* genotyping in women with weak D could facilitate better evaluation of appropriate candidates for RhIG administration,[44] and algorithms have been published to select appropriate patients for *RHD* genotyping.[45,46]

Postpartum Prevention of Alloimmunization to the D Antigen

All D-negative females who deliver D-positive infants should receive at least a 300-μg dose of IM or IV RhIG unless previous maternal immunization to the D antigen, not related to antepartum RhIG therapy, has been demonstrated. If the result of the infant's typing is questionable, RhIG should be given to the mother. A postpartum maternal blood sample must be drawn and evaluated for the extent of FMH. If the screening test for FMH is positive (FMH screen will detect over 30 mL of fetal red cell contamination), hemorrhage must be quantified to assess the need for additional doses of RhIG. This is usually accomplished by performing a Kleihauer-Betke test or a flow-cytometric assay. A full dose (300 μg) of RhIG protects against alloimmunization to the D antigen after exposure of up to 15 mL of D-positive red cells (or 30 mL of whole blood). In about 1 in 300 deliveries, the FMH exceeds 15 mL of red cells, and one or more additional doses of RhIG are required. In this setting, IV RhIG may prove to be a convenient alternative to multiple IM injections. RhIG should be administered to the mother within 72 hours of delivery. However, if more than 72 hours have elapsed, the dose should still be given, as it may still protect against maternal alloimmunization. Antepartum administration may cause a positive antibody screen in the mother because of passively acquired antibody. Antepartum RhIG has been associated with a weakly reactive direct antiglobulin test result in the newborn, but this is not associated with clinical evidence of hemolysis. Obtaining a careful patient history is essential in determining the likely cause of anti-D in the pregnant or postpartum female. Because administration of anti-D to D-negative individuals carries minimal risk, RhIG should always be given when there is any question about whether the anti-D is caused by passive or active immunization. (See also Chapter 4: Transfusion Practices.)

Special Considerations

The package insert should be followed carefully for determination of dose for any indication. RhIG may also be used when D-positive blood components are given to D-negative females of childbearing potential and to children. A 300-µg dose is sufficient to protect against the immunizing effect of the D-positive red cells contained in platelet products, although this practice may not be necessary for a single dose of D-positive apheresis platelets.[47] The administration of multiple vials of RhIG after the transfusion of a full unit of D-positive red cells is generally impractical and probably unnecessary, given that D alloimmunization is uncommon in the trauma setting.[48] Some have advocated the use of red cell exchange transfusion in addition to IV RhIG when large amounts of D-positive red cells have been transfused to a D-negative recipient.

IV RhIG is approved by the FDA for use in D-positive patients with ITP who have not undergone splenectomy.[49] IV RhIG is an important alternative to IM therapy in patients with coagulopathy and significant thrombocytopenia. The initial dose is 50 to 75 µg/kg unless the hemoglobin level is less than 10 g/dL, in which case 25 to 40 µg/kg is recommended. Depending on the initial response, additional doses may be required. The response to anti-D may be related to *RHD* zygosity, with hemizygous *RHD* patients responding with higher platelet increases than homozygous *RHD* patients.[50] The primary advantages of IV RhIG over IVIG in the treatment of ITP are the lower cost and lower volume of IV RhIG. Risks of RhIG in ITP include red cell hemolysis, renal failure, and disseminated intravascular coagulation, and patients should be closely monitored.[51]

References

1. Medical and Scientific Advisory Council. MASAC recommendations concerning products licensed for the treatment of hemophilia and other bleeding disorders. MASAC Document 249. New York: National Hemophilia Foundation, 2017.
2. Franchini M. Systematic review of the role of FVIII concentrates in inhibitor development in previously untreated patients with severe hemophila A: A 2013 update. Semin Thromb Hemost 2013;39:752-66.
3. Peyvandi F, Mannucci PM, Garagiola I, et al. A randomized trial of factor VIII and neutralizing antibodies in hemophilia A. N Engl J Med 2016;374:2054-64.
4. Carcao M. Changing paradigm of prophylaxis with longer acting factor concentrates. Haemophilia 2014;20:99-105.
5. Mancuso ME, Santagostino E. Outcome of clinical trials with new extended half-life FVIII/IX concentrates. J Clin Med 2017;6:39.
6. Uchida N, Sambe T, Yoneyama K, et al. A first-in-human phase 1 study of ACE910, a novel factor VIII–mimetic bispecific antibody, in healthy subjects. Blood 2016;127:1633-41.
7. Montgomery RR, Gill JC, Scott JP. Hemophilia and von Willebrand disease. In: Nathan DG, Orkin SH, Ginsburg D, et al, eds. Nathan and Oski's hematology of infancy and childhood. 7th ed. vol. 2. Philadelphia: WB Saunders, 2009:1547-76.
8. Franchini M, Mannucci PM. Von Willebrand factor (Vonvendi): The first recombinant product licensed for the treatment of von Willebrand disease. Expert Rev Hematol 2016;9:825-30.
9. Kruse-Jarres R, Kempton CL, Baudo F, et al. Acquired hemophilia A: Updated review of evidence and treatment guidance. Am J Hematol 2017;92:695-705.

10. Shapiro A. Plasma-derived human factor X concentrate for on-demand and perioperative treatment in factor X-deficient patients: Pharmacology, pharmacokinetics, efficacy and safety. Expert Opin Drug Metab Toxicol 2017;13:97-104.
11. Sarode R, Milling TJ, Refaai MA, et al. Efficacy and safety of a 4-factor prothrombin complex concentrate in patients on vitamin K antagonists presenting with major bleeding: A randomized, plasma-controlled, phase IIIb study. Circulation 2013;128:1234-43.
12. Sorensen B, Spahn DR, Innerhofer P, et al. Clinical review: Prothrombin complex concentrates–evaluation of safety and thrombogenicity. Crit Care 2011;15:201-10.
13. Milling TJ, Refaai MA, Goldstein JN, et al. Thromboembolic events after vitamin K antagonist reversal with 4-factor prothrombin complex concentrate: Exploratory analyses of two randomized, plasma-controlled studies. Ann Emerg Med 2016;67:96-105.
14. Siegal DM, Garcia DA, Crowther MA. How I treat target-specific oral anticoagulant-associated bleeding. Blood 2014;123:1152-8.
15. Pollack CV, Reilly PA, Eikelboom J, et al. Idarucizumab for dabigatran reversal. N Engl J Med 2015;373:511-20.
16. Menache D, Grossman BJ, Jackson CM. Antithrombin III: Physiology, deficiency and replacement therapy. Transfusion 1992;32:580-8.
17. Maclean P, Tait RC. Hereditary and acquired antithrombin deficiency. Drugs 2007;67:1429-40.
18. Grottke O, Henzler D, Rossaint R. Activated recombinant factor VII (rFVIIa). Best Pract Res Clin Anaesthesiol 2010;24:95-106.
19. Stanworth SJ, Birchall J, Doree CJ, et al. Recombinant factor VIIa for the prevention and treatment of bleeding in patients without haemophilia. Cochrane Database Syst Rev 2007;(2):CD005011.
20. Levi M, Levy JH, Andersen HF, Truloff D. Safety of recombinant activated factor VII in randomized clinical trials. N Engl J Med 2010;363:1791-800.

21. Spotnitz WD, Burks S. Hemostats, sealants, and adhesives II: Update as well as how and when to use the components of the surgical toolbox. Clin Appl Thromb Hemost 2010; 16:497-514.
22. Albala DM, Lawson JH. Recent clinical and investigational applications of fibrin sealant in selected surgical specialties. J Am Coll Surg 2006;202:685-97.
23. Franchini M, Lippi G. Acquired factor V inhibitors: A systematic review. J Thromb Thrombolysis 2011;31:449-57.
24. Rea CJ, Foley JH, Ingerslev J, Sorensen B. Factor XIII combined with recombinant factor VIIa: A new means of treating severe haemophilia A. J Thromb Haemost 2011; 9:510-16.
25. Tahlan A, Ahluwalia J. Factor XIII. Arch Pathol Lab Med 2014;138:278-81.
26. Moldovan D, Bernstein JA, Cicardi M. Recombinant replacement therapy for hereditary angioedema due to C1 inhibitor deficiency. Immunotherapy 2015;7:739-52.
27. The SAFE Study Investigators. A comparison of albumin and saline for fluid resuscitation in the intensive care unit. N Engl J Med 2004;350:2247-56.
28. Perel P, Roberts I, Ker K. Colloids versus crystalloids for fluid resuscitation in critically ill patients. Cochrane Database Syst Rev 2013;(2):CD000567.
29. Larsson SJ, Bragadottir G, Krumbholz V, et al. Effects of acute plasma volume expansion on renal perfusion, filtration, and oxygenation after cardiac surgery: A randomized study of crystalloid vs. colloid. Br J Anaesth 2015;115: 736-42.
30. Pagano MB, Harmon MC, Cooling L. Use of hydroxyethyl starch in leukocytapheresis procedures does not increase renal toxicity. Transfusion 2016;56:2848-56.
31. Knezevic-Maramica I, Kruskall MS. Intravenous immune globulins: An update for clinicians. Transfusion 2003;43: 1460-80.
32. Römer J, Morgenthaler JJ, Scherz R, et al. Characterization of various immunoglobulin preparations for intravenous

application 1. Protein composition and antibody content. Vox Sang 1982;42:62-73.
33. Schwab I, Nimmerjahn F. Intravenous immunoglobulin therapy: How does IgG modulate the immune system? Nat Rev Immunol 2013;13:176-89.
34. Kotlan B, Stroncek DF, Marincola FM. Intravenous immunoglobulin-based immunotherapy: An arsenal of possibilities for patients and science. Immunotherapy 2009; 1:995-1015.
35. Anderson D, Ali K, Blanchette V, et al. Guidelines on the use of intravenous immune globulin for hematologic conditions. Transfus Med Rev 2007;21(Suppl 1):S9-S56.
36. Alejandria MM, Lansang MA, Dans LF, Mantaring JB. Intravenous immunoglobulin for treating sepsis, severe sepsis, and septic shock. Cochrane Database Syst Rev 2013;(9):CD001090.
37. Cowden J, Parker SK. Intravenous immunoglobulin production, uses and side effects. Pediatr Infect Dis J 2006; 25:641-2.
38. Gelfand EW. Intravenous immune globulin in autoimmune and inflammatory diseases. N Engl J Med 2012;367:2015-25.
39. Cunningham-Rundles C, Zhou Z, Mankarious S, et al. Long-term use of IgA-depleted intravenous immunoglobulin in immunodeficient subjects with anti-IgA antibodies. J Clin Immunol 1993;13:272-8.
40. Pierce LR, Jain N. Risks associated with the use of intravenous immunoglobulin. Transfus Med Rev 2003;17:241-51.
41. American College of Obstetricians and Gynecologists. Prevention of Rho(D) isoimmunization. ACOG Practice Bull 1999;4:1-8. (ACOG-reaffirmed 2013.)
42. Hartwell EA. Use of Rh immune globulin: ASCP practice parameter. Am J Clin Pathol 1998;110:281-92.
43. Bowman J. Thirty-five years of Rh prophylaxis. Transfusion 2003;43:1661-6.
44. Sandler SG, Roseff SD, Domen RE, et al. Policies and procedures related to testing for weak D phenotypes and

administration of Rh immune globulin: Results and recommendations related to supplemental questions in the comprehensive transfusion medicine survey of the College of American Pathologists. Arch Pathol Lab Med 2014;138: 620-5.
45. Sandler SG, Flegel WA, Westhoff CM, et al. It's time to phase in RHD genotyping for patients with a serologic weak D phenotype. Transfusion 2015;55:680-9.
46. Clarke G, Hannon J, Berardi P. Resolving variable maternal D typing using serology and genotyping in selected prenatal patients. Transfusion 2016;56:2980-5.
47. Bartley AN, Carpenter JB, Berg MP. D+ platelet transfusions in D– patients: Cause for concern? Immunohematology 2009;25:5-8.
48. Dutton RP, Shih D, Edelman BB, et al. Safety of uncrossmatched type-O red cells for resuscitation from hemorrhagic shock. J Trauma 2005;59:1445-9.
49. Sandler SG, Tutuncuoglu SO. Immune thrombocytopenic purpura–current management practices. Expert Opin Pharmacother 2004;5:2515-27.
50. Despotovic JM, McGann PT, Smeltzer M, et al. RHD zygosity predicts degree of platelet response to anti-D immune globulin treatment in children with immune thrombocytopenia. Pediatr Blood Cancer 2013;60:E106-8.
51. Despotovic JM, Lambert MP, Herman JH, et al. RhIG for the treatment of immune thrombocytopenia: Consensus and controversy. Transfusion 2012;52:1126-36.

HEMOSTATIC DISORDERS

Overview of Hemostasis

Hemostasis refers to the physiologic mechanisms that control bleeding. Normal hemostasis may be viewed as occurring in three overlapping stages. Primary hemostasis involves blood vessels (particularly the endothelial layer) and cellular blood elements (particularly platelets) and culminates in the formation of the platelet plug. Secondary hemostasis involves plasma procoagulant proteins (clotting or coagulation factors) and the formation of a stable fibrin clot. The third stage involves repair of vascular damage that results in a return to the normal state. Two control processes, the fibrinolytic system and the anticoagulant system (consisting of inhibitor proteins and endothelial-cell-based mechanisms), are important in limiting clot formation to areas of vascular injury. Pathologic bleeding or thrombosis may result from derangement in either of these processes.[1]

Blood Vessels

Under normal circumstances, vascular endothelium maintains a thromboresistant surface by a variety of mechanisms, including secretion of the platelet inhibitory substances (such as prostacyclin and nitric oxide), expression of molecules involved in the inhibition of coagulation (eg, heparan sulfate and thrombomodulin), and provision of a barrier between intravascular elements and the tissue-factor-rich extravascular structures. After injury, the blood vessel constricts, which limits blood flow. The interaction of blood elements with subendothelial structures allows adhesion and activation of platelets, and activation of procoagulant mechanisms.

Hereditary blood vessel disorders associated with a bleeding diathesis include connective tissue disorders (eg, Ehlers-Danlos and Marfan syndromes) and vascular malformations (eg, hereditary hemorrhagic telangiectasia syndrome and giant hemangioma).

Acquired blood vessel disorders include medical conditions such as scurvy and vasculitis, vascular anomalies such as angiodysplasia, and physical disruptions such as those occurring with trauma or surgery. If available, treatment is directed to the underlying vascular abnormality. Postoperative anatomic bleeding caused by inadequate surgical hemostasis may be difficult to diagnose, particularly in patients with concomitant abnormalities of platelets or coagulation factors. In general, bleeding from one site suggests an anatomic lesion, whereas small-vessel bleeding from multiple sites (eg, wound edges, intravenous access sites, and the endotracheal tube) suggests abnormal hemostatic mechanisms.

Platelets

Platelets are anuclear cell fragments produced by megakaryocytes under the influence of cytokines such as thrombopoietin; they function to form a cohesive plug at the site of vessel injury. Endothelial disruption results in exposure of blood elements to extravascular collagen and tissue factor (TF). Platelet interaction with collagen—either directly via platelet glycoprotein VI (GPVI) or indirectly through adhesion to immobilized von Willebrand factor via platelet GPIb/IX—leads to platelet capture. Platelet adhesion drives multiple secondary processes, including activation of the platelet fibrinogen receptor (GPIIb/IIIa) and release of platelet granular contents, leading to aggregation of more platelets to the growing hemostatic plug. Platelets play an important role in the coagulation system as well. Coagulation proteins and Ca^{++} are stored within platelet granules, and coagulation factors assemble on the phospholipid surface of activated platelets, localizing thrombin generation.[2] In addition, platelets can influence leukocyte trafficking, inflammation, response to sepsis, tissue regeneration, and angiogenesis.[3]

Coagulation Proteins

The initial platelet plug that forms at a site of vascular injury is stabilized by fibrin generated by the coagulation mechanism, a closely regulated series of reactions. The coagulation mechanism consists of procoagulant serine proteases that circulate as zymogens (ie, Factors II, VII, IX, X, XI, and XII), nonenzymatic cofactors (ie, Factors V and VIII), the substrate for fibrin gel formation (fibrinogen), and fibrin-stabilizing enzymes [Factor XIII and thrombin-activatable fibrinolysis inhibitor (TAFI)]. Coagulation can be divided into three phases: initiation, amplification/propagation, and clot formation.[2]

In vivo, the exposure of TF to blood is the key step in the initiation of coagulation.[4] TF is abundantly present in the subendothelium, may be expressed on activated endothelial cells (and possibly synthesized by activated platelets), and may also be transported to sites of vascular injury in the form of circulating microparticles. TF triggers the coagulation system at the site of injury by capturing circulating Factor VIIa. The Factor VIIa-TF complex converts Factor X to its active form either directly or indirectly via activation of Factor IX. Phospholipid-membrane-bound Factor Xa then forms a complex with Factor Va, which in turn converts the zymogen prothrombin to the active enzyme thrombin. This thrombin functions in the amplification/propagation phase by feedback activation of Factors XI, VIII, and V. This positive feedback sustains further thrombin generation after the Factor VIIa-TF process is inhibited by TF pathway inhibitor (TFPI). Inadequate amplification of the initial hemostatic signal is thought to explain why hemophiliacs bleed despite normal levels of Factor VII. The thrombin generated via the amplification/propagation mechanism performs multiple functions, including conversion of fibrinogen to fibrin clot, further activation of platelets through protease-activated receptors, and activation of Factor XIII. Factor XIIIa stabilizes the clot by covalent crosslinking of fibrin.

In vitro, coagulation can be initiated by another protease/cofactor system, the so-called contact factor system. Deficiencies of the contact factors (ie, Factor XII, prekallikrein, and kininogen) will prolong the activated partial thromboplastin time (aPTT) screening test (see below) but are not associated with a clinical bleeding diathesis.

Natural Anticoagulant Systems and Fibrinolysis

The processes by which procoagulant activities are limited to the site of injury are important in regulation of normal hemostasis. Two main processes are involved: the natural anticoagulant systems, which consist primarily of circulating and endothelial-based protease inhibitors, and the fibrinolytic system, which is primarily responsible for the proteolytic dissolution of the fibrin clot. Blood fluidity depends largely on the integrity of the two anticoagulant proteins, antithrombin and protein C. Antithrombin inhibits activated coagulation serine proteases, primarily thrombin and Factor Xa. Heparin and heparan-like molecules markedly augment antithrombin activity. Protein C is activated by thrombin bound to thrombomodulin on endothelial cells. Activated protein C, in the presence of protein S, degrades Factors Va and VIIIa. The protein C system subserves both anticoagulant and anti-apoptotic/anti-inflammatory functions. A mutation in Factor V (Factor V Leiden) results in resistance to the anticoagulant action of activated protein C and increased risk of venous thrombosis.[5]

Fibrinolysis is accomplished by the enzyme plasmin, which is formed by the action of endothelial-cell-based activators upon its circulating zymogen, plasminogen. Fibrin serves as a cofactor in its own degradation. In the presence of fibrin, endothelial-cell-released tissue plasminogen activator (tPA) converts plasminogen to plasmin. Plasmin binds to the newly formed fibrin and breaks it down to soluble degradation products, which leads to clot lysis.[6] Unbound plasmin can also degrade fibrinogen, Factor V, and Factor VIII. In-vivo regulation of plasmin activity occurs at three levels: 1) plasminogen activator inhibitor (PAI-1) blocks the activation of plasminogen by inhibiting plasminogen activators, 2) alpha$_2$-plasmin inhibitor inhibits plasmin, and 3) in the presence of thrombomodulin, thrombin can activate TAFI, which in turn decreases the susceptibility of fibrin clot to lysis. An increased level of plasminogen activator, a deficiency of PAI, or a deficiency of alpha$_2$-plasmin inhibitor may each cause a bleeding tendency through increased plasmin activity. Conversely, derangement of the fibrinolytic mechanisms (such as elevated PAI-1 levels or dysfibrinogenemia) may increase thrombotic risk.

Evaluation of Bleeding Disorders

Personal and family history may be the most important "screening investigation" in the evaluation of a patient with a history of bleeding. Mucosal bleeding (epistaxis, menorrhagia, gastrointestinal bleeding), excessive bruising, or bleeding after minor trauma or immediately after surgery is suggestive of either a defect of platelets or von Willebrand disease (vWD). Bleeding into joints, muscles, or soft tissues suggests a coagulation factor deficiency, such as hemophilia. Delayed bleeding may suggest a deficiency of Factor XIII or the inhibitors of fibrinolysis. Diseases associated with disturbances of hemostasis include liver disease, renal disease, malabsorptive syndromes, disorders of the marrow, and sepsis. Medications may inhibit platelet function, decrease platelet number, or interfere with vitamin K metabolism.

Physical examinations should evaluate the size and distribution of sites of bleeding. Petechiae are characteristic of severe thrombocytopenia, while ecchymosis is nonspecific. Significant lymphadenopathy, hepatomegaly, or splenomegaly may indicate malignancy or hepatic disease. Hyperflexibility may indicate a collagen disorder, such as Ehler-Danlos syndrome. However, bleeding does not necessarily indicate an intrinsic defect of hemostasis, as bleeding will occur in the setting of a normal hemostatic mechanism in the face of sufficient challenge (trauma, surgery, etc).

Laboratory evaluation of the platelet component of hemostasis is routinely assessed by two screening methods: the platelet count and platelet function assessment. Evaluation of platelet hemostatic function in a patient with a history of bleeding symptoms remains difficult.[7] The platelet function analyzer (PFA-100, Siemens, Deerfield, IL) closure time has largely replaced the bleeding time test; the closure time reported is the time required for platelets and plasma proteins in a patient's whole-blood sample to generate an obstructive aggregate at an aperture of a collagen-coated membrane.[8] The PFA-100 assay detects relatively severe defects, including abnormalities of platelet adhesion (eg, vWD or Bernard-Soulier syndrome), abnormalities of platelet secretion (eg, storage pool defect, aspirin effect, etc) and disorders of aggregation (eg, Glanzmann thrombasthenia). A platelet count under 80,000/µL and hemoglobin level under 10 g/dL often prolongs the closure time. Because of suboptimal sensitivity and specificity, PFA-100 is generally not recommended as a screen for milder forms of vWD and milder platelet function defects.[9] A patient with a significant history of bleeding in the face of an adequate platelet count and normal coagulation screening (see below) merits evaluation for vWD (with assays of vWF antigen, vWF activity, and Factor VIII level) and/or a platelet function disorder (with assays such as platelet aggregation studies). Finally, it is worth noting that the PFA-100 assay lacks the sensitivity or specificity to be used as a routine preoperative screening tool, nor does it replace a detailed clinical history in the evaluation of the risk of surgical bleeding.[8]

Laboratory screening of coagulation includes 1) the prothrombin time (PT, which evaluates the extrinsic pathway: Factors VII, X, V, and II, and fibrinogen); 2) the activated partial thromboplastin time (aPTT, which evaluates the intrinsic pathway: contact factors; Factors XI, IX, VIII, X, V, and II; and fibrinogen); and 3) either the thrombin time (TT, which evaluates the fibrinogen-to-fibrin conversion step and is sensitive to the effect of heparin) or a quantitative fibrinogen assay. Interpretation of the PT and aPTT should be taken in context. Acquired mild-to-moderate prolongation of the PT that results from liver disease is often not associated with significant increase in bleeding risk, probably because of concomitant reductions in proteins C and S.[10] However, in congenital hemostatic disorders (such as mild hemophilia), minor abnormalities of the PT or aPTT may be indicators of a clinically significant coagulation factor deficiency. Therapeutic levels of the coagulation factors required for hemostasis and the indications for factor replacement depend upon the patient's clinical status and the magnitude of the hemostatic challenge. Conversely, a normal aPTT does not exclude a diagnosis of mild hemophilia. Thrombin generation assays are an additional global test of coagulation, but such assays remain research rather than clinical tools. Coagulation factor levels above 25% to 35% and fibrinogen levels above 100 to 150 mg/dL are generally sufficient to prevent major hemorrhage,[11,12] but higher levels may be desirable for patients facing major surgery or with trauma-related bleeding.[13,14]

If symptoms of delayed bleeding are present, Factor XIII assay and evaluation of fibrinolysis may be indicated. Laboratory markers of an activated fibrinolytic system are not readily available,[14] but a shortened euglobulin clot lysis time (<60 minutes) suggests a hyperfibrinolytic state. A decrease in the plasma fibrinogen level or an elevation of TT, fibrin degradation products, or D-dimer may also point to activated fibrinolysis. Severe liver disease and hepatic surgery (resection or transplantation) are the most common causes of primary fibrinolysis.

Whole blood viscoelastic monitoring of the hemostatic mechanism has been gaining acceptance in both monitoring of the hemostatic mechanism and guidance of transfusion therapy.[15] (See Chapter 5: Patient Blood Management for detail.) Viscoelastic tests such as thromboelastography (TEG) and rotational thromboelastometry (ROTEM) assess global coagulation and clot dynamics in real time, through the phases of initiation of clotting, clot formation, and potentially clot lysis.[16] They are performed on whole blood, yielding initial results within minutes, and the assays are generally completed within 30 to 60 minutes. Viscoelastic monitoring has been investigated in conjunction with therapeutic algorithms in multiple settings, including antithrombotic therapy for coronary artery disease (TEG platelet mapping[17]), extracorporeal membrane oxygenation,[18] massive transfusion,[19] and surgery.[20,21]

Platelet Disorders

Thrombocytopenia

Many conditions can result in thrombocytopenia.[22] When it results from marrow suppression (from radiation, chemotherapy, nutritional deficiency, or toxic drugs), platelet transfusions are usually successful in elevating the platelet count and lowering the bleeding risk. In nonbleeding patients with thrombocytopenia caused by marrow failure, prophylactic platelet transfusions are generally reserved for platelet counts below 10,000/µL.[23,24] Although clinical factors such as fever, sepsis, splenomegaly, renal failure, or drugs (eg, amphotericin) have been used to justify a higher threshold (ie, 20,000/µL), the effectiveness of that strategy has been questioned.[23] However, transfusion thresholds over 10,000/µL have been advocated for patients on anticoagulation therapy, for patients who have had a recent and severe bleeding episode, and for neonates. Response to prophylactic platelet transfusion should be assessed to help guide continued therapy and to detect platelet refractoriness. (See Chapter 1: Blood Components; Chapter 4: Transfusion Practices.) Multiple factors may result in decreased responsiveness to platelet transfusion.[25] In addition to disease-related factors [such as splenomegaly, sepsis, fever, disseminated intravascular coagulation (DIC), or complications of hematopoietic stem cell transplantation], patients who have been repeatedly transfused or pregnant may develop antibodies to HLA or platelet-specific antigens that are present on the platelet surface. Such patients may respond to transfusion of HLA- or crossmatch-selected products. (See Management of Platelet Refractoriness, Chapter 4.) In patients who are refractory to platelet transfusion despite these measures, antifibrinolytic therapy may be useful.[26]

In patients who are actively bleeding or who are about to undergo major nonneuraxial invasive procedures, platelet transfusions are often indicated for counts below 50,000/μL.[22-25] Platelet counts as high as 100,000/μL may be desired for support of patients requiring extracorporeal membrane oxygenation (ECMO)[27] and procedures in which any increased bleeding would be problematic, such as neurologic surgery.[22,23] AABB has published a consensus guideline for minor procedures, suggesting that a platelet count of over 20,000/μL is sufficient for safe insertion of a central venous catheter, and over 50,000/μL is safe for lumbar puncture.[24]

In contrast, accelerated destruction of peripheral blood platelets (because of consumptive or immune disorders) is more difficult to treat with transfusions because the transfused platelets are rapidly destroyed. For this reason, transfusion to increase the platelet count is generally not undertaken in autoimmune thrombocytopenia; however, transfusion may be useful in the management of acute hemorrhage in these patients.[25,28] Reports of disease exacerbation and mortality statistics suggest that platelet transfusions are hazardous in patients with thrombotic thrombocytopenic purpura (TTP) or heparin-induced thrombocytopenia (HIT).[29] These patients should receive platelet transfusion only when it is medically necessary for control of active bleeding.[30,31]

Platelet Function Defects

Platelet function defects may be congenital or acquired.[7,32] Congenital disorders include abnormalities of platelet granules or membrane receptors, and include defects of adhesion (eg, Bernard-Soulier syndrome due to deficiency of GPIb/IX or platelet-type vWD), defects of platelet aggregation (eg, Glanzmann thrombasthenia due to deficiency of GPIIb/IIIa), or defects of platelet metabolism or granular content (eg, gray platelet syndrome, dense granule deficiency). Acquired disorders are most often caused by drugs, especially aspirin, nonsteroidal anti-inflammatory agents, and platelet receptor antagonists (thienopyridines and GPIIb/IIIa inhibitors). Patients with uremia and those undergoing procedures involving extracorporeal circulation may have platelet function defects.[33]

Desmopressin (DDAVP) has been reported to be effective in treating bleeding associated with both uremia and congenital platelet function abnormalities.[33] DDAVP releases Factor VIII and vWF from endothelial cells and other storage sites, but other mechanisms may also be contributing to the therapeutic effect (See Prohemostatic Drugs, below, for details of administration.) Response to DDAVP in a patient with a platelet function defect is empirically assessed; there is no convincing evidence that laboratory monitoring is useful. Platelet transfusion can be used to treat selected platelet function defects, but the hemostatic defect seen with uremia will not respond to platelet transfusion alone. Treatment of bleeding in uremic patients without thrombocytopenia includes dialysis, maintenance of the hematocrit >30%,[32] administration of DDAVP, and conjugated estrogens. For some patients, systemic or topical administration of antifibrinolytic therapy may be appropriate. Finally, recombinant Factor VIIa (rFVIIa, NovoSeven, NovoNordisk, Princeton, NJ) has proven effective for controlling bleeding in patients with Glanzmann thrombasthenia, a licensed indication for the treatment in the United States.[33]

Aspirin is a mild platelet antagonist that inhibits platelet thromboxane production, whereas thienopyridines (eg, clopidogrel and prasugrel) and ticagrelor (a nucleoside analogue) inhibit the platelet adenosine diphosphate (ADP) receptor. Aspirin and clopidogrel are irreversible inhibitors of platelet function. Recommendations for delaying surgery for patients on these agents varies depending on the indications for which the medications are being administered, the surgical bleeding risk, and the interval between surgery and the patient's last dose of medication.[13] Assessment of platelet function may provide guidance as to whether prophylactic platelet transfusion is necessary in situations where surgery cannot be postponed.[13] GPIIb/IIIa inhibitors (eg, abciximab, eptifibatide, and tirofiban) are potent inhibitors of platelet aggregation that block the GPIIb/IIIa receptor for fibrinogen and vWF. They also inhibit thrombin generation and platelet procoagulant activity and prolong the activated clotting time. These drugs significantly reduce thrombotic complications in patients with acute coronary syndromes who are undergoing percutaneous coronary intervention.[34] Platelet function returns to about half the pretreatment status in about 4 to 12 hours depending on the drug given.[35] Patients who develop bleeding after receiving the longer-acting GPIIb/IIIa inhibitor abciximab may require repeated platelet transfusions to counteract the effect of the drug. Thrombocytopenia is an infrequent complication of GPIIb/IIIa inhibitor therapy and is seen in less than 1.0% of cases.[36] Discontinuation of the GPIIb/IIIa inhibitor is recommended with thrombocytopenia, and in severe cases, platelet transfusion may be appropriate.

Congenital Bleeding Disorders

von Willebrand Disease

vWD is a very common hereditary bleeding disorder[37] that may result from quantitative or qualitative abnormalities of vWF.

vWF is a large multimeric molecule that is secreted from endothelial cells, is present in both plasma and platelets, and mediates platelet adhesion to subendothelial tissues at sites of vascular injury. Platelet plug formation is defective in patients with vWD. Another vWF function is as a chaperone for coagulation Factor VIII. Diminished Factor VIII levels are frequently seen in patients with more severe forms of vWD. Regulation of vWF function is complex, and the metalloprotease ADAMTS13 is involved in preventing formation of inappropriate vWF-platelet microthrombi. (See Thrombotic Microangiopathies, on page 45.)

vWD manifests most commonly as mucosal bleeding, but deep tissue bleeding can occur in severe cases. A diagnosis of vWD is confirmed by specific assays of both vWF and Factor VIII.[38] Because of the multiplicity of vWF defects, a classification system has been adopted (See Table 5). The most common form of vWD is mild-to-moderate quantitative vWF deficiency (Type 1 vWD), which is generally attributable to decreased production of vWF; however, in rare individuals, quantitative deficiency results from increased vWF clearance (Type 1C). For patients in whom production of vWF is virtually absent (Type 3 vWD), Factor VIII levels are in the same range as those in patients with moderate hemophilia A. Type 3 vWD is inherited as an autosomal recessive disorder, but the condition can be mimicked in rare individuals on an autoimmune basis. While Types 2A, 2B, and 2M vWD are all attributable to structural defects of vWF that undermine the interaction of vWF with platelets, patients with Type 2N vWD manifest unexpectedly low Factor VIII levels as a result of impaired transporter function of vWF. Finally, there are multiple forms of acquired vWD, a condition that is becoming more commonly recognized as a complication with the use of left ventricular assist devices for patients with congestive cardiomyopathy.[40]

DDAVP (desmopressin) is primarily useful to increase vWF levels and restore hemostatic function in patients with Type 1 vWD. DDAVP is not useful in patients with severe (Type 3) disease. The utility of DDAVP in the qualitative variants (Types

Table 5. Classification, Bleeding Phenotype, and Treatment of Bleeding in vWD*

Type	Description	Bleeding Phenotype	Treatment of Choice†	Alternative Treatment
1 (including 1C)	Partial quantitative deficiency of vWF	Mild to moderate	DDAVP	Intermediate-purity Factor VIII concentrate Recombinant vWF
2	Qualitative defect of vWF			
2A	Decreased vWF-dependent platelet adhesion with selective deficiency of high-molecular-weight multimers	Usually moderate	Intermediate-purity Factor VIII concentrate Recombinant vWF	DDAVP
2B	Increased vWF affinity for platelet GPIb	Usually moderate	Intermediate-purity Factor VIII concentrate Recombinant vWF	Platelet transfusion is indicated if thrombocytopenia persists after vWF replacement

(Continued)

Table 5. Classification, Bleeding Phenotype, and Treatment of Bleeding in vWD* (Continued)

Type	Description	Bleeding Phenotype	Treatment of Choice[†]	Alternative Treatment
2M	Decreased vWF-dependent platelet adhesion with no multimer defects	Usually moderate	Intermediate-purity Factor VIII concentrate Recombinant vWF	DDAVP
2N	Markedly decreased vWF binding to Factor VIII	Usually moderate	Intermediate-purity Factor VIII concentrate	DDAVP
3	Virtually complete deficiency of vWF (manifests as severe Factor VIII deficiency)	Severe bleeding	Intermediate-purity Factor VIII concentrate Recombinant vWF	Platelet transfusion; if patient has alloantibodies, recombinant Factor VIII or VIIa

*Modified from Nichols et al[37] and Breakey.[39]
[†]Adjuvant treatment with antifibrinolytics is recommended for mucosal bleeding for all types of vWD.
vWD = von Willebrand disease; vWF = von Willebrand factor; DDAVP = desmopressin; GP = glycoprotein.

2A, 2M, and 2N) is patient specific and less predictable. DDAVP is relatively contraindicated in individuals with qualitative variants characterized by increased interaction between vWF and platelets (Type 2B and the rarer platelet-type vWD caused by mutations of platelet GPIb), because DDAVP administration may worsen thrombocytopenia in those patients. DDAVP is usually given in doses of 0.3 µg/kg intravenously over 20 minutes, but it is also available as a concentrated nasal spray (Stimate, CSL Behring, King of Prussia, PA). Administration of an elective test dose is helpful to confirm a patient's responsiveness, and most patients with Type 1 vWD experience a twofold to fivefold increase of vWF levels 30 to 60 minutes after administration. DDAVP-induced elevation of vWF levels generally persists for about 8 to 10 hours,[37,38] but the response may be significantly shorter in patients with increased clearance (Types 1C and 2A) and patients with acquired vWD.

Tachyphylaxis may develop; thus DDAVP may not be effective after three or four consecutive daily doses.[41] Mild and transient side effects include headache and facial flushing. To prevent hyponatremia and water retention caused by the antidiuretic effect of DDAVP, patients should restrict fluid intake for 24 hours after DDAVP administration. DDAVP should be used with caution in elderly individuals with cardiovascular disease and in children weighing <20 kg. Pregnancy is not a contraindication for DDAVP; however, its use may complicate fluid management. Furthermore, many patients with Type 1 vWD will experience an increase in vWF levels by the end of pregnancy sufficient that they can undergo parturition without requiring additional support of the vWF level.[37]

Patients who are unresponsive to DDAVP or have Type 2B and Type 3 variants require exogenous vWF-containing factor concentrate. Intermediate-purity plasma-derived products contain both vWF and Factor VIII: Humate-P (CSL Behring), Alphanate (Grifols Biologicals, Los Angeles, CA), and Wilate (Octapharma, Vienna, Austria). They are labeled in both vWF ristocetin cofactor activity units (vWF:RCo units) and Factor

VIII units. Recently, recombinant vWF (Vonvendi, Shire, Westlake Village, CA) has been approved by the Food and Drug Administration (FDA); that product does not supply Factor VIII. High-purity Factor VIII concentrates prepared by monoclonal or recombinant technology are devoid of vWF and should not be used for treatment of vWD. Although Cryoprecipitated AHF contains both Factor VIII and vWF, its use in the treatment of vWD (or hemophilia A) should be reserved for urgent situations when virus-attenuated factor concentrates are not immediately available. Cryoprecipitated AHF is not quality assured for vWF content, and reports suggest that it contains approximately 90 to 170 vWF:RCo units per individual unit of Cryoprecipitated AHF.[42]

Dosage of vWF-containing concentrate is calculated by determining the desired increment of vWF level and taking into account the recovery of infused protein. (See Table 6 for dose calculations and Table 7 for recommended target vWF levels.) For life-threatening bleeding or major surgery, a recommended initial target vWF:RCo level of 80% to 100% is suggested, and follow-up therapy is aimed at preserving hemostatic levels for at least 3 days. However, recommendations for the duration of factor support vary widely between surgical procedures.[37] For minor bleeding episodes, a single dose chosen to achieve a vWF:RCo level of 40% to 50% may be sufficient. In a patient with Type 2N vWD (in which the Factor VIII levels are lower than vWF levels because of an abnormal interaction of Factor VIII with vWF) or Type 3, replacement therapy is more complicated. For treatment of Type 2N vWD, the recommended replacement concentrate must contain vWF. However, the dose calculations should be based on the product's labeled Factor VIII activity by using calculations appropriate for Factor VIII replacement. (See sections on hemophilia.) Support of both the vWF and Factor VIII level is required during the initial management of Type 3 vWD, and dose calculations should take both hemostatic proteins into account. In Type 3 vWD, if bleeding persists despite adequate levels of vWF and Factor VIII, transfusion of platelets to transport vWF to areas of injury may be effective.[43] Approximately 10% to 15% of

Table 6. Calculations of Doses of Factor Concentrate

Definitions

1. **Target level**: Level of factor desired for a given clinical situation. (See Table 8.)
2. **Desired increment**: Rise in factor level desired to increase factor level from the preinfusion level to the target level (measured in IU/dL, %, or mg/dL).
3. **Weight**: Patient's weight in kilograms.
4. **Recovery** is established by the concentrate manufacturer, empirically determined and generally listed in the product insert as unit/dL increase per unit/kg administered to the patient. Check product insert for exact recovery data.
- Factor VIII: ~2 IU/dL per IU/kg infused
- Factor IX: ~0.76 to 1 IU/dL per IU/kg infused
- Factor X: ~2 IU/dL per IU/kg infused
- von Willebrand factor: ~1.5 IU/dL per IU/kg infused
- Antithrombin (plasma-derived): ~1.4 IU/dL per IU/kg infused
- Protein C (plasma-derived): ~1.4 IU/dL per IU/kg infused
- Fibrinogen (plasma-derived): ~1.7 mg/dL per IU/kg infused

Calculation of Dose

Dose = (desired increment × weight)/recovery

Note: Dose, frequency, and duration of therapy are dependent upon the severity of the deficiency, age, and clinical situation of the patient. Recovery varies between recombinant preparations, and values listed above are approximate. See text and package inserts of the various factor preparations for further details.

patients with Type 3 vWD develop antibodies that inactivate vWF or cause anaphylactic reactions. Bleeding in these patients may respond to treatment with either high doses of recombinant Factor VIII or rFVIIa.[43]

Antifibrinolytic therapy is an important adjunctive therapy for patients with vWD and is useful for treatment of bleeding in mucosal areas that are rich in fibrinolytic activity. Lysine analogues (epsilon aminocaproic acid and tranexamic acid) interfere with plasmin binding to fibrin, thereby inhibiting fibrinolysis. These medications are contraindicated in upper urinary tract bleeding because urinary tract obstruction may result from failure of clot lysis.[43]

Hemophilia A—Factor VIII Deficiency

Hemophilia A is an X-linked congenital bleeding disorder caused by Factor VIII deficiency. Gene deletions, gene rearrangements, and point mutations of the Factor VIII gene have been described.[11] The clinical severity of hemophilia is related to a patient's factor level. Severe hemophiliacs (defined as baseline Factor VIII levels below 1%) are at risk for spontaneous hemorrhage. Moderate hemophiliacs have Factor VIII levels of between 1% and 5% and may have excessive bleeding with minimal trauma or after surgery, whereas patients with factor levels above 5% are considered mild hemophiliacs, in whom significant trauma usually precedes bleeding episodes.

Unlike platelet-related bleeding, hemophilic bleeding manifests spontaneously or several hours after the causative trauma and occurs most frequently in deep structures such as joints and muscles. Bleeding may occur anywhere, however, including in the brain and the gastrointestinal tract.

Similar to vWD, mild hemophilia A may be treatable with DDAVP if the patient is known to achieve a satisfactory post-DDAVP factor level, and the same principles of therapy apply.[1,11] Moderate or severe disease (and life-threatening bleeding episodes in patients with mild hemophilia A) requires factor-replacement therapy with Factor VIII concentrates. Recombinant Factor VIII concentrates have traditionally been considered the products of choice, but concern related to inhibitor development has spurred renewed interest in virus-inactivated plasma-derived Factor VIII.[44] (See Chapter 2: Plasma Derivatives.) Cryoprecipitated AHF is used only in urgent situations when preferred concentrates are not immediately available. Unlike the situation for vWF, the FDA requires that each unit of Cryoprecipitated AHF contain at least 80 international units (IU) of Factor VIII, but the actual content varies among facilities. The duration of factor-replacement therapy and target factor levels are dictated by the specific indications for treatment, severity of bleeding, and the patient's response to treatment.[1,11] For examples of target values for various indications, see Tables 7 and 8; more complete recommendations are available elsewhere. Hemophilic joint bleeding is typically treated with Factor VIII replacement to a target level of 40% to 80%, and a follow-up infusion given the next day with the aim of achieving a follow-up increment of 40%. In preparation for surgery or when replacement therapy is required for management of a life-threatening event, the desired Factor VIII level is at least 100% of normal. After initial replacement, follow-up therapy is provided to maintain trough Factor VIII levels above 50%. The average half-life of the majority of currently available Factor VIII products is approximately 8 to 12 hours, so maintenance factor support may be accomplished by providing a dose of Factor VIII sufficient to provide a 50% increment every 12 hours. Recently, several novel recombinant Factor VIII products with a somewhat longer half-life have been approved by the FDA, potentially allowing a longer interdose replacement interval.[11] Factor concentrate is occasionally administered as continuous infusion. Although this requires use of reconstituted product beyond the manufacturer's recommended limit, several studies have shown that Factor VIII administered in this fashion is stable for 24 to 72 hours.[45] Continuous infusion therapy allows for more stable factor levels and simplifies monitoring while also using less concentrate. Infusion is typically initiated at approximately 4 IU/kg/hour, and the dose is then titrated based on laboratory monitoring.[45]

Factor products are available as lyophilized concentrate. The quantity of Factor VIII coagulant activity is stated on the vial label in IU. One IU is the amount of Factor VIII coagulant activ-

Table 7. Recommendations for Factor Replacement Therapy for Bleeding or Surgery in vWD*

Type of Surgery or Bleeding	Initial Dose[†‡] (vWF:RCo)	Subsequent Dose[†] (vWF:RCo)	Target vWF:RCo and Factor VIII Activity Trough[‡]
Minor (Gingival surgery, central line placement, complicated dental extraction, superficial biopsy, tonsillectomy, laparotomy)	30-60 U/kg	20-40 U/kg every 24-48 hours	>30-50 IU/dL for 1-5 days[§]
Major (Cardiothoracic surgery, caesarian section, craniotomy, open cholecystectomy, gastrointestinal surgery)	40-60 U/kg	20-40 U/kg every 8-12 hours	>50 IU/dL for 7-14 days[§]

*Modified from Nichols et al.[37]
[†]DDAVP should be used as first-line treatment if appropriate.
[‡]To avoid risk of thrombosis, vWF:RCo should not exceed 200 IU/dL, and Factor VIII should not exceed 250-300 IU/dL.
[§]Because of vWF's early role in hemostasis, maintenance of adequate Factor VIII levels becomes more important after the first 2 to 3 days.
vWD = von Willebrand disease; DDAVP = desmopressin; vWF:RCo = von Willebrand ristocetin cofactor.

Table 8. Initial Target Factor Levels for Various Clinical Situations (units/dL) and Half-Life of Infused Material

Clinical Situation	Factor VIII	Factor IX	vWF
Life-threatening bleeding or surgery	80-100	80-100	80-100
Hemophilic joint bleeding	60-100	60-100	NA
Minor bleeding event	20-40	20-40	30-40
Half-life (hours)	10-19	15-92	8-19

Note: Target level and frequency of follow-up doses should be decided according to the clinical situation, factor half-life, and other clinical variables.[11,37]
vWF = von Willebrand factor; NA = not available.

ity present in 1 mL of normal plasma. The method of calculation for dosing that is generally used by hematologists involves the empiric observation that each unit of Factor VIII infused per kilogram of body weight yields a 2% rise in the plasma Factor VIII activity level (ie, 0.02 IU/mL or 2 IU/dL). In hospitalized patients who require repeated infusions, the Factor VIII levels should be monitored to ensure adequate replacement.

Approximately 10% to 15% of patients with severe hemophilia A develop neutralizing immunoglobulin G (IgG) antibodies after repeated Factor VIII infusions.[11] These patients with inhibitors require therapeutic products that have Factor-VIII-bypassing activity. (See Management of Inhibitors to Factor VIII or Factor IX, below.) Acute management of hemophilic bleeding is best managed in conjunction with an experienced consultant who is familiar with the care of this condition.

Hemophilia B—Factor IX Deficiency

The inheritance and clinical manifestations of Factor IX deficiency are identical to those of Factor VIII deficiency. Although the principles of replacement therapy are similar for these disorders, several specific differences must be pointed out. DDAVP and Cryoprecipitated AHF are *not* effective in the treatment of patients with Factor IX deficiency; replacement therapy for patients with hemophilia B requires the infusion of products that contain Factor IX. Although concentrates are available from either plasma-derived or recombinant sources, most hemophilia treatment centers in the United States rely on recombinant materials. Dosing schedules for Factor IX vary from that for Factor VIII, because of the differences in the two factors' hemostatic effectiveness, volume of distribution, and half-life. (See Tables 6 and 8.) In the initial treatment of hemophilic joint hemorrhage, the target Factor IX level is 30% to 60%, and the follow-up dose administered the next day is targeted to achieve an increment of 30%. In preparation for surgery or when replacement therapy is required for the management of a life-threatening event, the desired Factor IX level is at least 80% of normal. After initial replacement, follow-up therapy is provided to maintain trough Factor IX levels above 40%. The calculation for dosing of Factor IX concentrate is based on determining the desired increment in Factor IX concentration required for the particular clinical situation, the weight of the patient, and the recovery of the specific Factor IX concentrate chosen for replacement therapy. (See Tables 6 and 8 for calculation.) The average half-life of infused non-half-life-extended Factor IX products is approximately 15 to 24 hours; 82 to 101 hours have been reported for genetically engineered or glycoPEGylated extended-half-life recombinant Factor IX preparations.[11,46] Factor levels should be monitored in patients who require sustained factor levels, as is required after surgery or severe bleeding episodes.

Approximately 1% to 4% of hemophilia B patients develop inhibitors (antibodies) to Factor IX. These antibodies generally develop early in their clinical history and may be associated with anaphylactic reactions.[47] A bleeding hemophilia B patient with an inhibitor may respond to bypassing agents. (See Management of Inhibitors to Factor VIII or Factor IX, below.)

Management of Inhibitors to Factor VIII or Factor IX

Development of inhibitory antibodies to a coagulation factor is a serious consequence of factor-replacement therapy for hemophilia. The potency of inhibitors is generally reported in Bethesda units (BU). Patients with low titers of inhibitors (<5 BU) may achieve satisfactory responses to increased doses of factor, but this approach is generally fruitless in patients with higher-titer inhibitors. Immune tolerance therapy, aimed at eradication of the inhibitor antibody through daily infusions of high doses of Factor VIII or IX, has been successful in producing tolerance in up to 70% of hemophilia A patients but in only 30% of hemophilia B patients.[11,47]

Factor products that possess "bypassing activity," such as activated prothrombin complex concentrates (aPCCs) or rFVIIa,[47-49] are the mainstay of therapy for patients with inhibitors. The precise mechanism of action of an aPCC (such as FEIBA-NF, Shire, Westlake Village, CA) is unclear, but evidence points to the activation of Factor X and prothrombin, which bypasses the role of Factors VIII and IX in the coagulation mechanism. The initial dose of 50 to 100 units/kg can be repeated in 6 to 12 hours, but thrombotic complications have been reported with repeated use of aPCCs. Concurrent use of antifibrinolytics should therefore be avoided with this agent. The primary mechanisms of action of rFVIIa appear to involve TF-dependent activation of Factor X and TF-independent activation of Factors IX and X on the surface of activated platelets. The licensed recommended dose is 90 µg/kg, but more recent investigations have explored the use of doses as high as 270 µg/kg. In the treatment of inhibitor patients, rFVIIa has had few adverse side effects and a low risk of thrombosis.[50] Drawbacks of using bypassing agents include expense, absence of a laboratory monitor for treatment efficacy, and a short plasma half-life (estimated at 2.7 hours for rFVIIa). No therapy is universally successful in the management of hemophilia patients with inhibitors, and consultation with a physician experienced in patient care in these challenging situations is prudent.

In rare instances, spontaneous Factor VIII inhibitors occur as an autoimmune process in previously normal individuals. These autoantibodies are mainly seen in the postpartum setting or in elderly patients with associated autoimmune or malignant disease. Patients usually present with severe bleeding. Patients with autoantibody to Factor VIII generally have a low titer of cross-reactivity to porcine Factor VIII and often will respond to treatment with recombinant porcine factor (Obizur, Shire, Westlake Village, CA).[51,52] Alternatively, acute bleeding episodes may be managed in a fashion similar to that for hemophilia patients with inhibitors through the use of rFVIIa or aPCCs. Immunotherapy aimed at suppression of autoantibody is used for long-term control in these patients.[53] Inhibitors to other coagulation factors occur very rarely.

Factor XI Deficiency

In Factor XI deficiency, the bleeding tendency varies widely among individuals and is poorly correlated with factor level. Mucosal bleeding and menorrhagia are the most frequent presenting symptoms. Diagnosis may be complicated by the fact that many aPTT assays are insensitive to mild Factor XI deficiency; if this disease is suspected, specific measurement of Factor XI is suggested. Although extensive hemorrhage can occur after trauma or surgery, some patients have tolerated surgery without excessive bleeding despite an almost undetectable Factor XI level; an individual patient's history of clinical bleeding in comparison to hemostatic challenge should be reviewed as one decides whether there is a need for factor replacement before a surgical procedure. Factor XI concentrate is not available in the United States, and treatment with plasma to achieve a Factor XI level 30% to 45% of normal is sufficient for hemostasis in most situations. Factor XI has a half-life of 52 ± 22 hours. Low-dose rFVIIa has also been used off-label in this setting. DDAVP and antifibrinolytic agents may be important adjunctive therapies.[12,54]

Other Congenital Factor Deficiencies

Deficiencies of vitamin-K-dependent Factors II, VII, or X and deficiency of the non-vitamin-K-dependent Factors V and XIII are rare causes of congenital bleeding diathesis.[12] (See Table 9.) With the notable exceptions of Factor XI (discussed above) and Factor VII, the severity of bleeding manifestations is generally correlated with a patient's measured factor level.

rFVIIa is the replacement product of choice for treatment of congenital Factor VII deficiency.[12] Although the half-life of rFVIIa is about 3 hours, doses of 15 to 30 μg/kg administered at intervals of 4 to 6 hours have been successful. For both Factors II and X, a level of approximately 30 IU/dL is generally considered sufficient for surgery. A plasma-derived Factor X concentrate is available (Coagadex, Bio Products Laboratories, Elstree, UK) with a recovery of 2.1 IU/dL for each unit/kg infused, and a mean postinfusion half-life of 30 hours.[55] Alternative replacement products that might be used in an urgent situation could include plasma or PCC. Plasma [Fresh Frozen Plasma, Thawed Plasma, Plasma Frozen Within 24 Hours After Phlebotomy (PF24), etc] is commonly chosen for replacement therapy in patients with deficiency of Factor II, but PCCs or Octaplas (Octapharma, Vienna, Austria) could be considered as a virus-attenuated alternative. PCCs contain variable amounts of all of the vitamin-K-dependent factors, and a physician should know the factor content of the PCC preparation that is being considered. There is a paradoxical risk for thrombosis when PCCs are used, and monitoring of both factor levels and DIC markers is recommended should repeated doses of PCC be used.

For patients with congenital deficiency of the non-vitamin-K-dependent Factor V, preoperative levels of 25% to 30% are recommended. Plasma is the treatment of choice for replacement of Factor V, with a loading dose of 15 to 20 mL/kg followed by 3 to 6 mL/kg every 24 hours as necessary to maintain factor levels. The half-life of infused Factor V is approximately 36 hours.[12] Although Factor V is called "labile factor," it is only minimally decreased in PF24 or Thawed Plasma.[56,57]

Table 9. Clinical Features and Management of Bleeding of the Rare Coagulation Disorders*

Deficient Factor	Main Clinical Symptoms	Hemostatic Levels	Plasma Half-Life	Recovery (as % of amount infused)	Treatment
Fibrinogen (hypo- and afibrinogenemia)	Umbilical cord, joint, and mucosal bleeding; bruising; major hemorrhage from birth trauma; surgical bleeding	100-150 mg/dL	2-4 days	50%	Cryoprecipitate (goal fibrinogen level 80-100 mg/dL initially) Fibrinogen concentrate Fibrin sealant
Prothrombin	Umbilical cord, joint, and mild mucosa bleeding; surgical bleeding	10%-30%	3-4 days	40%-80%	PCC Plasma
Factor V	Mucosal bleeding, surgical bleeding, moderately severe bleeding in homozygotes	10%-20%	36 hours	80%	Plasma Platelets

Factor	Symptoms	Level	Half-life	Target level	Treatment
Factor VII	Mucosal, joint (may be severe), and muscle bleeding; surgical bleeding; levels may correlate poorly with bleeding symptoms	15%-20%	4-6 hours	70%-80%	Recombinant Factor VIIa 4-Factor PCC Plasma
Factor X	Epistaxis/mucosal, umbilical cord, joint, and muscle bleeding; surgical bleeding	20%-40%	30-40 hours	50%	Factor X concentrate PCC Plasma
Factor XI	Posttraumatic bleeding (variable bleeding with different surgeries), epistaxis	15%-20%	40-50 hours	90%-100%	Plasma
Factor XIII	Umbilical cord, intracranial, and joint bleeding; recurrent miscarriages; surgical bleeding; impaired wound healing	2%-5%	9-12 days	—	Cryoprecipitate Factor XIII concentrate

(Continued)

Table 9. Clinical Features and Management of Bleeding of the Rare Coagulation Disorders* (Continued)

Deficient Factor	Main Clinical Symptoms	Hemostatic Levels	Plasma Half-Life	Recovery (as % of amount infused)	Treatment
Factors V + VIII	Mucosal bleeding, surgical bleeding	15%-20%	36 hours for Factor V and 10-19 hours for Factor VIII	60%-80%	Plasma and recombinant Factor VIII concentrate for severe deficiency
Vitamin-K-dependent factors	Umbilical cord and intracranial bleeding; surgical bleeding	15%-20%	See corresponding factors	—	Vitamin K1 (phytomenadione) 4-factor PCC Plasma

*Modified from Peyvandi and Menegatti,[12] and Xavier et al.[54]
PCC = prothrombin complex concentrate.

Patients with congenital Factor XII deficiency have no bleeding symptoms despite their having a prolonged aPTT, and do not require replacement therapy.

Severe Factor XIII deficiency is a bleeding disorder that often presents with umbilical stump bleeding. It is also associated with a high risk of spontaneous intracranial hemorrhage. PT, aPTT, and fibrinogen assays are normal, and specific tests of Factor XIII function will confirm a diagnosis. Replacement is achieved with pasteurized plasma-derived concentrate (Corifact, CSL Behring, King of Prussia, PA) or, in appropriate patients, a recombinant Factor XIII A-subunit preparation (Tretten, Novo Nordisk, Plainsboro, NJ).[58] Although Cryoprecipitated AHF also contains Factor XIII,[42] it is no longer the preferred replacement but would be acceptable in an urgent setting should the above-mentioned products be unavailable.[12,54] Factor XIII has a long half-life (5-11 days). Levels should be maintained above 5% to 10% to prevent spontaneous intracranial hemorrhage, but higher levels (at least 10% to 25%) are suggested for surgery.

Inherited disorders of fibrinogen may be quantitative or qualitative. In patients with congenital defects, fibrinogen replacement therapy may be indicated to treat or prevent surgical bleeding, improve wound healing, or prevent recurrent pregnancy loss. The FDA has licensed a heat-treated fibrinogen concentrate (RiaSTAP, CSL Behring) for patients with congenital fibrinogen deficiency, while Cryoprecipitated AHF remains the only FDA-licensed product for use in other settings.[42,59] Fibrinogen has a long half-life (55-120 hours) and suggested minimum target levels are 50 mg/dL to prevent recurrent pregnancy loss, and over 100 to 150 mg/dL in surgical settings.[54] However, in settings of consumptive hypofibrinogenemia, as occurs with complications of pregnancy or trauma, levels over 150 to 200 mg/dL are recommended.[60]

Alpha$_2$-Plasmin Inhibitor

Deficiency of alpha$_2$-plasmin inhibitor, the primary circulating plasmin inhibitor, is associated with a severe hemorrhagic disorder. Diagnosis requires a specific assay for this inhibitor. Therapy consists of replacement by plasma transfusion and/or oral antifibrinolytic agents such as epsilon aminocaproic acid (EACA).[61]

Acquired Bleeding Disorders

Vitamin K Deficiency and Vitamin K Antagonists

Vitamin K is a fat-soluble vitamin that is necessary for synthesis in the liver of coagulation Factors II, VII, IX, and X; protein C; and protein S. Nutritional deficiency states can occur in patients in the intensive care unit, those who have chronic disease and are receiving antibiotics, and those with general fat-malabsorption states, such as celiac disease, pancreatic insufficiency, or obstructive jaundice. The dose and route of vitamin K administration depend on the clinical situation. Oral administration is preferred over subcutaneous administration because of the delayed and unpredictable response to subcutaneously administered vitamin K.[62] Historically, intravenous infusion of vitamin K has been associated with anaphylaxis, but a slow infusion rate reduces the risk for patients in whom the oral route is unavailable. The full effect of vitamin K is achieved only after 12 to 24 hours; thus, urgent correction of deficiencies of the vitamin-K-dependent factors requires factor infusion in addition to vitamin K replacement (see below).

Vitamin K antagonists such as warfarin are still commonly used for outpatient anticoagulation therapy, interfering with the vitamin-K-dependent synthesis of coagulation Factors II, VII, IX, and X. Despite their effectiveness, vitamin K antagonists are plagued with problems, including a narrow therapeutic window, considerable dose-response variability between patients, interactions with both drugs and dietary factors, and difficulty in maintaining a therapeutic degree of anticoagulation [as monitored by the international normalized ratio (INR)]. In rare cases, warfarin-induced skin necrosis can develop about 1 to 4 days after initiation of therapy, which is related to the drug's early effect on protein C synthesis. Patients with congenital deficiency of protein C or its cofactor (protein S) are at increased risk for the development of this complication of warfarin therapy and may warrant coverage with heparin-based therapy until the full warfarin effect is achieved. Warfarin overdose is treated by withdrawal of the drug and/or the administration of vitamin K. In the absence of bleeding, 0.5 to 2 mg of oral vitamin K may be sufficient, but 2.5 mg or higher doses are recommended. The optimal dose of vitamin K has not been evaluated through clinical trials.[62] Urgent replacement of vitamin-K-dependent coagulation factors is addressed below.

Other Anticoagulant Drugs: Heparins and Directed Oral Anticoagulants

Heparin-based drugs [either conventional unfractionated heparin (UFH) or lower-molecular-weight derivatives] are among the most frequently prescribed medications to treat or prevent thromboembolism. Heparin markedly enhances the ability of antithrombin to neutralize serine proteases. Even slight contamination of a diagnostic sample with UFH (eg, the flush volume in a subclavian catheter) can prolong the TT and the aPTT, which can lead to confusion in diagnosis. The risk of bleeding in patients taking heparin drugs is modified by many factors, including comorbid conditions (such as recent surgery, trauma, or renal failure), the patient's age and gender, and the use of concomitant antiplatelet drugs.[63] UFH therapy is monitored by either using the aPTT or by directly assessing heparin activity via the anti-Factor Xa assay. Plasma is not effective in reversing heparin effect, and acute UFH reversal is accomplished with protamine sulfate.[64] At the completion of cardiac bypass surgery, algorithms or point-of-care instruments can be used to estimate the quantity of circulating heparin in order to select an appropriate protamine dose; 1 mg of protamine sulfate neutralizes 80 to 100 units of UFH. Protamine has a shorter half-life than UFH, and "rebound" heparin effect or initial underestimation of the protamine dose should be considered in a patient with unexplained bleeding after protamine therapy.[41] Low-molecular-weight heparin (LMWH) is derived by enzymatic or chemical depolymerization of UFH. FDA-approved indications and dose schedules differ between the various approved LMWH preparations, but as a class they share most attributes. LMWH drugs have less anti-Factor IIa activity (and therefore less effect on the aPTT) than does UFH, but they retain the ability to accelerate antithrombin effect against Factor Xa, and thus they remain potent anticoagulant drugs. Compared to UFH, LMWH produces a more predictable anticoagulant response, has a longer plasma half-life (3 to 12 hours), and fewer interactions with osteoclasts and platelets. These qualities translate into weight-based dosing on a once- to twice-daily time frame, no need to monitor levels in most patient settings, and a reduced risk for HIT. The aPTT is not an appropriate monitor of LMWH effect, and specific drug levels (via anti-Factor Xa assay) are required if monitoring is desired. LMWH is cleared mainly through a renal mechanism, and dose adjustment is required in patients with significant renal impairment. If excessive bleeding occurs, protamine may be helpful but is not a completely effective antidote.

Fondaparinux (Arixtra, GlaxoSmithKline, Research Triangle Park, NC) is a synthetic pentasaccharide that strongly binds antithrombin and acts as a selective inhibitor to Factor Xa. It is administered parenterally, has a half-life of 17 to 21 hours, and is cleared primarily through renal excretion. Clinical licensing has been for thromboprophylaxis in the orthopedic setting and for initial treatment of venous thrombotic disease; dose schedules are weight-based and do not rely on drug level monitoring. Fondaparinux is not neutralized by protamine and is not easily removed via dialysis. Case reports suggest that off-label use of rFVIIa has been helpful in patients who develop severe bleeding complications while on fondaparinux.[65]

Direct-acting coagulation factor inhibitors can be classified as parenterally administered, short-acting agents or direct-acting oral anticoagulants (DOACs). The two parenterally administered direct thrombin inhibitors have been available for several years.[66] Argatroban (GlaxoSmithKline, Research Triangle Park, NC) is a competitive inhibitor of thrombin and is most often used in the setting of HIT. It is administered by continuous infusion and has a plasma half-life of approximately 45 minutes, but clearance is very prolonged in patients with hepatic dysfunction (even if this is caused by passive congestion after cardiac surgery). Bivalirudin (Angiomax, The Medicines Co., Parsippany, NJ) is a recombinant peptide drug based on the amino acid sequence of hirudin, the anticoagulant protein present in the salivary secretions of the medicinal leech. Bivalirudin binds to thrombin reversibly and has a short plasma half-life (approximately only 25 minutes). Bivalirudin is partially cleared by the kidney, and the remaining clearance occurs via proteolysis. It is indicated for treatment during acute coronary angioplasty and in unstable angina. Given their short half-lives, bleeding complications that arise during the use of these two direct thrombin inhibitors is handled by drug discontinuation and general hemostatic measures.[64]

DOAC medications are becoming established as attractive alternatives to vitamin K antagonists. The advantages of these agents over other agents for chronic anticoagulation management include their oral route of administration, predictable dose response, rapid onset of action, and fewer drug or dietary interactions than vitamin K antagonists. Clinical studies in orthopedic thromboprophylaxis, prevention of systemic thromboembolism in the setting of atrial fibrillation, and prevention of recurrent venous thromboembolic disease, have generally shown noninferiority or superiority compared with vitamin K antagonists or LMWH. Clinical laboratory monitoring of anticoagulant effect was not performed in these trials, and routine monitoring is not a recommended component of patient-care algorithms that use these agents. However, "on-therapy" drug levels have been reported, and either screening for the presence of these drugs (via

TT or anti-Factor Xa assay) or assessment of actual drug level may be useful in rare instances.[67] Dabigatran (Pradaxa, Boeringer Ingelheim, Ridgefield, CT) is an oral targeted thrombin inhibitor. Its half-life is 14 to 17 hours in patients with normal renal function, and dose modification is required in patients who have significant renal insufficiency. Routine coagulation tests are of limited value in assessing anticoagulant effect; however, the aPTT may be prolonged on therapy, and the TT is exquisitely sensitive in demonstrating that drug is present. Dabigatran effects are efficiently and immediately reversed by infusion of the monoclonal drug idarucizumab.[68,69] Rivaroxaban (Xarelto, Janssen Pharmaceutical, Titusville, NJ), apixaban (Eliquis, Pfizer, New York, NY), and edoxaban (Savaysa, Diiachi-Sankyo, Parsippany, NJ) are examples of oral targeted Factor Xa inhibitors. With a half-life of approximately 12 hours, these agents are metabolized by a combination of renal and hepatic mechanisms, and medication will accumulate if clearance mechanisms are impaired. The PT may be prolonged with rivaroxaban, but the anti-Factor Xa agents have no significant effect on the aPTT, and they do not prolong the TT. Before elective surgery, targeted oral anticoagulants should be discontinued for a sufficient interval to allow dissipation of drug effect. This interval should be adjusted based on the degree of renal function and surgical bleeding risk.[70] Routine coagulation assays with PT and aPTT may not be sensitive to confirm that a patient has cleared DOAC before surgery; however, a normal TT (dabigatran) or normal anti-Xa assay (rivaroxaban, apixaban, and edoxaban) suggests that the drug has been cleared. Reversal agents for the oral anti-Factor Xa agents [andexanet alfa (AndexXa, Portola Pharmaceuticals, San Francisco, CA) and ciraparantag (PER977, Perosphere, Danbury, CT)] are in clinical trials. There is no clinical evidence that plasma products will reverse the anticoagulant effect of target-specific oral anticoagulants, but preclinical studies suggest a potential role for PCC, rFVIIa, or aPCC.[64,69,70] (See section below.)

Management of Bleeding in Patients on Anticoagulant Drugs

Serious bleeding in a patient on anticoagulant therapy merits a systematic approach that begins with general nonpharmacologic measures.[69] These include assessing the clinical stability of the patient and bleeding source, documenting the time of the last dose of anticoagulant medication, interrupting further anticoagulant administration, evaluating preexisting renal and hepatic impairment in order to estimate the residual anticoagulant effect, and performing hematologic laboratory assessment (complete blood count, PT/INR, aPTT, fibrinogen, TT, and measure of antithrombotic effect of drug or drug level, if available). Application of physical methods to quell the bleeding source should be applied if possible (such as mechanical pressure; endoscopic or radiologic interventions, if necessary; or surgery). Appropriate measures should be taken to correct hemodynamic compromise with fluid resuscitation and red cell transfusion, if necessary. Pharmacologic measures to reverse or overcome the effects of anticoagulant medications should be included in patient care when appropriate.

For bleeding episodes in which either vitamin K deficiency or warfarin effect is a confounding issue, factor-replacement therapy may be required in addition to vitamin K administration. This can best be accomplished by infusion of 4-factor PCC (containing significant amounts of Factor VII in addition to Factors II, IX, and X; see Chapter 2: Plasma Derivatives).[64] PCC is generally labeled by its Factor IX content, and dosing algorithms of PCC have been proposed based on the patient's weight and INR.[71] In a setting where PCC is unavailable and urgent reversal of vitamin K antagonism is required, plasma can be administered; however, volume overload and time delays are common complications of such therapy.

Immediate and complete reversal of dabigatran effect is accomplished with intravenous administration of idarucizumab,[68] but until agents such as andexanet-alfa[72] and ciraparantag[73] become available, only nonspecific reversal strategies can be employed for treating urgent bleeding for patients taking rivaroxaban, apixaban, and edoxaban. The effectiveness of 4-factor PCC is difficult to assess from the current literature, but case reports describe the use of PCC in patients with major or life-threatening bleeding. In-vitro and animal model studies provide data to suggest that these agents may help override the anticoagulant effect of DOACs, but the use of such agents in bleeding patients is generally discouraged.[69]

Antiplatelet Agents

Application of antiplatelet drug therapy has expanded greatly, owing to an appreciation of the role of platelets in arterial thrombotic disease and a growing understanding of platelet physiology.[74] Aspirin has multiple favorable properties. For most patients, daily low-dose aspirin is sufficient to inhibit the action of platelet cyclooxygenase, providing platelet inhibition by preventing the generation of thromboxane A_2. Although aspirin does not completely inhibit platelet function, it has the advantages of the oral route, low expense, and the availability of vast clinical experience. Disadvantages include an estimated incidence of major gastrointestinal hemorrhage of 1 to 2 per 1000 patient-years and the recognition of interindividual variation in effectiveness ("aspirin resistance"). Metabolic derivatives of thienopyridine drugs such as clopidogrel (Plavix, Bristol-Myers Squibb/Sanofi Pharmaceuticals, Bridgewater, NJ) and prasugrel (Effient, Eli Lilly, Indianapolis, IN) selectively inhibit ADP-induced activation of platelets via irreversible alteration of the platelet P_2Y_{12} receptor. Similar to aspirin, thienopyridines are administered by daily oral dosing, which is sometimes initiated with a larger loading dose. The effect of clopidogrel and prasugrel lasts approximately 7 days. Ticagrelor (Brilinta, AstraZeneca, Wilmington, DE) is a potent but reversible P_2Y_{12} receptor inhibitor, although it too has an effect that lasts several days.[75] Although transfusion of platelets may seem rational for the treatment of patients on antiplatelet agents who experience intracranial hemorrhage, a recent prospective study suggested that the volume of hemorrhage was not reduced by such interventions, and that 3-month outcomes were poorer in transfused compared to nontransfused individuals.[76]

Inhibitors of platelet activation are only partially effective; a class of more potent platelet inhibitory drugs relies on interrupting the final common pathway of platelet aggregation via inhibition of the platelet fibrinogen receptor (GPIIb/IIIa). Abciximab (ReoPro, Eli Lilly) is a recombinant chimeric antibody fragment with a functional effect that lasts approximately 48 hours after infusion. Peptide analogues of the sequence of fibrinogen that bind GPIIb/IIIa include epifibatide (Integrilin, Merck, Kenilworth, NJ) and tirofiban (Aggrestat, Merck). Epifibatide (a cyclic heptapeptide) and tirofiban (a peptidomimetic drug) have a short plasma half-life, and drug infusions are used if continued prolonged platelet inhibition is required. Bleeding complications that occur during use of the glycoprotein receptor-inhibiting drugs are best managed by a multidisciplinary team after assessment of the risks and benefits of intervention. In addition to general hemostatic measures, drug cessation should be considered. Platelet transfusion (two adult doses) should be considered as an additional measure for critical bleeding or to prevent bleeding in the rare patient who develops severe thrombocytopenia as a complication of the use of GPIIb/IIIa antagonist drugs.[64,77]

Liver Disease

Patients with liver disease have multiple coagulation derangements, including coagulation factor deficiencies, impaired vitamin K utilization, and activated fibrinolysis. Thrombocytopenia may add to the bleeding diathesis, and it is usually the result of multiple factors that include hypersplenism, increased platelet consumption, and diminished hepatic thrombopoietin production. However, parallel to the reduction in procoagulants, there is a reduction of physiologic control proteins including protein C, protein S, antithrombin, and ADAMTS13, and an increase in vWF level, together suggesting a "rebalancing" of hemostatic mechanisms at a new level.[78] How these hemostatic abnormalities influence the risk and severity of bleeding related to operative procedures or complications of portal hypertension is unclear. In patients with liver disease and laboratory indicators of abnormal synthesis of coagulation factors, vitamin K supplementation should be considered.[22] Liver biopsy, paracentesis, and thoracentesis are common diagnostic procedures in patients with liver disease, but there is a paucity of data to suggest that mild abnormalities of INR predict periprocedural bleeding.[79] Furthermore, correction of the INR is often not accomplished with the volume of plasma product infused.[80] Data are scarce regarding the threshold for platelet transfusion before liver biopsy; some institutions use 50,000/μL.[81] Viscoelastic testing provides a more global assessment of the hemostatic mechanism compared to INR and platelet count, and the results of viscoelastic testing suggest that transfusion therapy may be unnecessary in many patients with cirrhosis undergoing invasive procedures.[82] Alternative approaches to reduce the risk of bleeding with liver biopsy include using a transvenous approach, or "plugging" after biopsy. It is important to note that patients with hepatic failure may require larger volumes of plasma than do other patients to achieve PT improvement. Patients with liver disease and mild coagulopathy are sensitive to dilutional coagulopathy. The optimal strategy for the management of the bleeding liver disease patient remains to be defined. Although plasma (10-20 mL/kg) is reasonable in bleeding liver disease patients to prevent dilution of coagulation factors with the infusion of replacement red cells or plasma-free solutions, the use of coagulation factor concentrates, such as 4-factor PCC, has been suggested in order to deliver a sufficient dose of procoagulant factors while avoiding fluid overload. The value of rFVIIa for decreasing the transfusion requirement in bleeding patients with cirrhosis has been explored in multiple settings, but well-conducted clinical trials have generally shown little advantage to the use of this approach.[83]

Disseminated Intravascular Coagulation

A multitude of disorders, including infections, malignancy, and inflammatory conditions, lead to activation of the coagulation mechanism. If the activation overwhelms compensatory mechanisms, the clinical syndrome of DIC manifests. Increased degradation of coagulation proteins and protease inhibitors and widespread microvascular thrombosis leads to depletion of coagulation proteins and platelets.[84] The diagnosis of DIC requires integration of both clinical and laboratory data. The chief clinical manifestation in the acute form of DIC is organ dysfunction, but bleeding or thrombotic events may also require clinical attention. Routinely employed laboratory tests are neither sensitive nor specific for diagnosis of DIC, and thus a panel of studies is usually needed to make the diagnosis. Serial measurement of PT, aPTT, platelet count, and fibrinogen level to identify progressive reduction in coagulation components is helpful to establish the diagnosis and guide therapy in this dynamically changing condition. Thrombocytopenia is present in 80% to 90% of cases, and D-dimer is elevated in 99%. Vigorous treatment of the underlying disease, correction of acidosis, and aggressive support of tissue perfusion are the cornerstones of therapy. In the bleeding patient (or one requiring an invasive procedure), the transfusion of platelets, plasma, and/or Cryoprecipitated AHF should be guided by clinical parameters and laboratory values. Specific thresholds for transfusion are not established, but maintaining a platelet count over 50,000/µL and a fibrinogen level over 150 mg/dL has been suggested.[22,85] If thrombosis and tissue ischemia are prominent, heparin may be used to inhibit thrombin generation, but such recommendations remain controversial.[22] Antithrombin concentrate has not been demonstrated to improve any clinically relevant endpoint. Potent antifibrinolytic or prohemostatic agents (such as EACA or rFVIIa) are generally not recommended in patients with DIC, as they theoretically could increase the thrombotic risk.[22]

Coagulopathy of Trauma and Massive Tissue Injury

Coagulopathy is a major contributor to mortality in patients who have incurred tissue injury related to trauma. Recent studies have revealed that while fluid resuscitation may contribute to coagulopathy, a major driver of trauma-induced coagulopathy is tissue hypoperfusion and release of histones or other materials from injured tissues, resulting in endothelial dysfunction. Maladaptive endothelial responses include increased activity of the thrombin/thrombomodulin axis with activation of protein C (aPC), resulting in both degradation of Factor V and Factor VIII and hyperfibrinolysis caused by inactivation of PAI-1 by aPC and potentially other proteases.[86] Protocols for "damage control resuscitation" have been developed at trauma centers. The goals of these programs are to improve hemostasis and stop bleeding, and to restore cardiac output and oxygen delivery to tissues. Minimizing crystalloid infusion and early infusion of plasma decreases the incidence of tissue edema and endothelial cell dysfunction in the trauma setting.[87] Mortality of trauma patients from uncontrolled hemorrhage has been reduced through initiation of "massive transfusion" protocols that include empiric hemostatic product support whereby transfusion of platelets and plasma is prescribed in a fixed ratio to red cell transfusion.[14,88] Despite the growing enthusiasm for massive transfusion protocols, the role of ongoing clinical assessment and laboratory monitoring to inform transfusion decisions should not be abandoned. Novel methods to improve laboratory turnaround time and communication have been described,[89] and viscoelastic testing (as described in Chapter 5: Patient Blood Management) has an established role in the trauma setting.[19,90] Thresholds for transfusion of platelets, plasma, and fibrinogen-containing concentrates are evolving, but expert panels have suggested maintaining a platelet count above 50,000 to 75,000/μL and a fibrinogen level above 100 to 150 mg/dL.[59,91] To avoid exacerbating hypothermia, blood components and fluids should be administered via a blood-warming device. Adjuvants to resuscitation in trauma-associated coagulopathy may include antifibrinolytics, such as tranexamic acid.[92,93] A controlled trial did not demonstrate a survival advantage of rFVIIa in the trauma setting.[94] Finally, the data from trauma settings are not generalizable to patients undergoing massive transfusion in other settings (such as massive bleeding that may complicate an elective surgical procedure) where hypotension, caused by volume loss, and massive tissue injury are less often comorbidities. Goal-directed therapy of coagulopathy that is guided by laboratory measures is suggested in that setting.[95] (See also Chapter 6: Blood Component Resuscitation in Trauma and Massive Bleeding.)

Prohemostatic Drugs

DDAVP is a synthetic analogue of vasopressin. Its mechanism of action as a prohemostatic agent is incompletely understood, but is mainly attributable to stimulation of the endothelial cells, with subsequent endothelial cell release of granular contents (vWF, Factor VIII, and tPA) and activation of nitric oxide synthetase. DDAVP has been used primarily in the treatment of mild inherited or acquired platelet function defects (eg, uremia), hemophilia A, and vWD (see earlier sections). It is usually administered intravenously at a dose of 0.3 µg/kg over 20 minutes or as a concentrated nasal spray designed for outpatient use (Stimate, CSL Behring). DDAVP has been studied as a tool for blood conservation in patients without underlying hemostatic defects undergoing elective cardiac or orthopedic surgery. Review of these studies fails to support the routine use of DDAVP in this setting, but it may be helpful in the subset of patients taking aspirin.[41,42]

The antifibrinolytic drugs that are available take the form of synthetic lysine analogues. EACA and tranexamic acid are synthetic lysine analogues. Through occupancy of lysine-binding sites of both plasminogen and the plasminogen activators, these agents delay clot resorption. Oral secretions are rich in plasminogen activators, and antifibrinolytic agents are useful as an adjunctive therapy in patients with bleeding disorders who require dental procedures; topical administration may provide therapeutic effect while avoiding systemic toxicities. The anhepatic phase of liver transplantation is another setting in which intense fibrinolysis may result in bleeding complications; studies support a therapeutic effect of antifibrinolytic agents in that setting. Antifibrinolytic agents have been shown to decrease blood loss in the cardiac surgery setting, and meta-analysis of studies confirmed both a decreased rate of surgical reexploration and decreased mortality in cardiac surgery patients.[13] Similarly, these medications might be considered for control of bleeding in patients requiring support with ECMO.[13] Other surgical settings where antifibrinolytic therapy has been associated with decreased bleeding include liver transplantation, partial hepatic resections, total joint replacement surgery, and trauma.[41,94] Antifibrinolytic agents have also been used in the management of thrombocytopenic bleeding (eg, immune thrombocytopenia and myelosuppressed patients refractory to platelet transfusion), but the results have been less consistent in thrombocytopenic patients.[41] Compared to EACA, tranexamic acid is six to 10 times more potent on a molar basis. Both drugs are water soluble, cleared through a renal mechanism, and have a relatively short half-life. The principal adverse effect of EACA is gastrointestinal intolerance, commonly presenting as nausea, cramps, or diarrhea. Hypotension may occur with rapid intravenous administration, and myopathy is a rare complication of prolonged use. Thrombosis has generally not been a complication of EACA use in the hemophilic or perioperative setting but is a significant risk in the setting of DIC.[41]

Conjugated estrogens have been used to augment hemostasis in a wide variety of settings, including uremia and patients with chronic bleeding associated with hereditary hemorrhagic telangiectasia or angiodysplasia. Administration of oral contraceptive is a first-line therapy for controlling menorrhagia in women with vWD. It is also used to prevent menorrhagia in women of childbearing potential undergoing myeloablative chemotherapy.[41]

Topical hemostatic agents are useful to control localized bleeding. A large array of materials are available. Topical compressive agents include oxidized regenerated cellulose and microfibrillar collagen. Anastomotic sealants contain thrombin, which may be compounded with fibrinogen and antifibrinolytics in the form of "fibrin glue."

Thrombotic Disorders

Thrombophilia is a term used by clinicians to describe venous or arterial thromboembolism that develops spontaneously, at an early age, or at an unusual site, or involves recurrent thrombotic events. It is multifactorial, and most thrombophilia patients have several acquired and genetic risk factors.[96] The list of currently recognized inherited thrombophilic defects includes deficiency of coagulation control proteins (ie, antithrombin, protein C, and protein S), subtle defects of coagulation control (eg, Factor V Leiden), and increased levels of coagulation factors (probably the mechanism underlying prothrombin G20210A). Elevation of homocysteine levels may involve both inherited and acquired factors. The list of acquired prothrombotic states is long, but it can be broken down into circumstantial factors (eg, advanced age, immobility, pregnancy, and hormone replacement therapy) and disease-related factors (eg, surgery, malignancy, presence of an intravascular device, antiphospholipid syndrome, and HIT). The most common manifestation is venous thromboembolic (VTE) disease, which presents as either deep vein thrombosis or pulmonary embolism. Thrombophilic defects also contribute to the risk of VTE recurrence, and their presence may be taken into account in planning the duration of long-term anticoagulation in patients who have experienced thrombosis. Patients with a history of symptomatic thrombophilia should be considered for thromboprophylaxis during periods of increased risk, such as surgery or pregnancy.[97]

Genetic and serologic evaluations of thrombophilia are not affected by anticoagulation, but tests of plasma coagulation factors are best delayed until the effects of acute thrombosis have passed and anticoagulation is completed. Antithrombin, protein C, and protein S levels may transiently decrease and fibrinogen and Factor VIII may increase in response to an acute thrombotic episode. Anticoagulant therapy complicates interpretation of assays used to evaluate thrombophilia, and such laboratory evaluations are best deferred in patients on active anticoagulant therapy. Heparin therapy may depress antithrombin levels. Warfarin therapy may also complicate interpretation of assays for lupus anticoagulant, and it suppresses protein C and protein S levels; protein S levels may not return to baseline for up to 4 to 6 weeks after discontinuing warfarin.[98] Direct oral anticoagulants interfere with assays of protein S activity and have varying effect in assays of antithrombin and protein C activity depending on the drug and the method for assessment. All anticoagulant drugs complicate interpretation of assays for lupus anticoagulant.[99]

Transfusion support of patients with thrombophilia is rarely required. However, replacement therapy might be considered in situations where anticoagulant drug therapy presents an unacceptable bleeding risk or is unsuccessful. (See below.)

Deficiency of Coagulation Control Proteins

Antithrombin is the most important protease inhibitor of activated coagulation factors and is central to the in-vivo effect of heparin-based anticoagulants. Both human-plasma-derived, virus-inactivated antithrombin concentrate (Thrombate III, Grifols, Research Triangle Park, NC) and recombinant antithrombin (Atryn, rEVO Biologics, Framingham, MA) are available. The recombinant material has a much shorter half-life, such that continuous infusion is recommended when that preparation is chosen. Replacement therapy is approved for treatment of patients with hereditary antithrombin deficiency in connection with surgery or parturition, when the risk of anticoagulant therapy may be considered unacceptable. Antithrombin replacement has also been used in settings where achievement of anticoagulation with heparin has proven difficult, but published evidence is limited.[13]

Heterozygous deficiencies of protein C and protein S, two vitamin-K-dependent anticoagulant proteins, are associated with recurrent thromboembolic disease. Homozygotes present with purpura fulminans as infants. Symptomatic patients are generally managed with anticoagulation. Initiation of warfarin anticoagulation is associated with an increased risk for development of warfarin-induced skin necrosis, and concomitant heparin therapy is suggested during this interval. Replacement therapy may be useful in some situations. Human-plasma-derived protein C concentrate (Ceprotin, Baxter Healthcare, Westlake Village, CA) is available for treatment and prophylaxis of patients with severe protein C deficiency presenting with purpura fulminans or venous thrombosis.[100]

Antiphospholipid Syndrome

Antiphospholipid antibody syndrome is a clinical entity in which patients present with symptoms of thrombosis (either arterial or venous), recurrent pregnancy loss, or thrombocytopenia, along with laboratory evidence of autoantibodies that appear targeted to a variety of phospholipid-binding proteins.[101] Although anticardiolipin is a clinically useful screening serologic assay, beta-2 glycoprotein I appears to be the specific antibody target. Prothrombin and annexin V are other potentially important antibody targets. Antiphospholipid antibodies also may interfere with the assembly of coagulation factors on phospholipid surfaces in vitro, manifesting as a coagulation inhibitor known as a lupus anticoagulant. The choice of the name *lupus anticoagulant* is unfortunate, because many of the patients with this entity do not have systemic lupus erythematosis and these antibodies are clinically associated with thrombosis. Laboratory diagnostic criteria for a lupus anticoagulant require 1) detection of a prolonged phospholipid-dependent coagulation time (usually both the aPTT and the dilute Russell viper venom time are tested); 2) incomplete correction of the prolonged clotting test by using a 1:1 mixture of patient plasma with normal plasma (demonstrating the presence of a coagulation inhibitor); and 3) correction of the prolonged clotting time upon addition of excess phospholipid (demonstrating phospholipid dependence). If the patient has clinical bleeding, then the absence of a specific factor deficiency or inhibitor should also be demonstrated. This last criterion is crucial because lupus anticoagulants are generally not associated with clinical bleeding unless prothrombin (Factor II) levels are also diminished (a diagnosis meriting evaluation if the PT is prolonged), and because Factor VIII inhibitors may confound interpretation of aPTT-based assays used to identify lupus anticoagulant.

Transfusion therapy for patients with antiphospholipid syndrome is rarely required. Situations where this might arise include surgical interventions or bleeding in patients with associated thrombocytopenia, or in patients with catastrophic antiphospholipid syndrome—a multiorgan failure syndrome associated with a high mortality rate in which treatment strategies include a combination of immune suppression, antithrombotic therapy, and therapeutic plasma exchange (TPE) [for which the syndrome is defined as American Society for Apheresis (ASFA) indication Category II].[102] Occasionally, bleeding is attributable to autoimmune prothrombin deficiency complicating antiphospholipid syndrome; in this setting, immune suppression is the principal intervention, but case reports suggest rFVIIa or plasma exchange may provide value in urgent settings.[103]

Heparin-Induced Thrombocytopenia

HIT is a drug-associated immune thrombocytopenic disorder characterized by paradoxical thrombosis. Diagnosis is a challenge, as both heparin-based thromboprophylaxis is being used more commonly in hospitalized patients and thrombocytopenia frequently complicates medical illness. The decline in platelet count generally occurs between days 4 and 14 of heparin-based therapy, decreasing to below 50% of the pretreatment level. Thrombotic risk is very high in this condition, and asymptomatic thrombosis should be considered in patients with HIT. Clinical scoring systems (such as the "4Ts" for magnitude of **T**hrombocytopenia, **T**iming of decrease in platelet count in relationship to when heparin exposure began, presence of **T**hrombosis, and exclusion of o**T**her causes for low platelet count) are useful, as a low score is helpful to exclude this disorder. Serologic studies for the presence of antibody to platelet factor 4/heparin complexes or platelet activation assays such as the serotonin release assay are used to confirm a diagnosis. If HIT is clinically suspected, heparin should be promptly discontinued, diagnostic evaluation should be initiated, and an alternative immediate-acting anticoagulant should be substituted to provide anticoagulation. Argatroban and bivalirudin are FDA-approved nonheparin anticoagulant medications for use in patients with HIT, but fondaparinux is increasingly being used in this condition, and DOACs are being explored.[30] Recent work suggests that intravenous immunoglobulin therapy may also have a therapeutic role in management of HIT.[104] Platelet transfusion is generally avoided in HIT, because bleeding complications are rare, and platelet transfusion may exacerbate the thrombotic tendency.[29]

Thrombotic Microangiopathies

Thrombotic microangiopathies (TMAs) are clinical syndromes characterized by widespread microvascular thrombosis resulting in consumptive thrombocytopenia, microangiopathic hemolytic anemia, and organ dysfunction. Distinction of the various disorders that present as TMA [including such diverse conditions as TTP, Shiga-toxin-associated hemolytic uremic syndrome (STEC-HUS), atypical hemolytic uremic syndrome (aHUS), DIC, severe hypertension, vasculitis, HELLP (hemolysis, elevated liver enzymes, low platelet count) syndrome, and complications of organ or hematopoietic stem cell transplantation] is important in order to allow initiation of the appropriate therapeutic intervention and to avoid the risks associated with institution of noneffective interventions.[105,106] TTP is characterized by severe ADAMTS13 deficiency (ADAMTS13 activity <5% to 10% activity), attributable to either inhibitory autoantibody or congenital deficiency. The presence of severe ADAMTS13 deficiency helps distinguish TTP from other thrombotic microangiopathies.[107] Treatment of TTP is considered a medical emergency, and TPE should be initiated immediately if TTP is clinically suspected. Delay in determination of ADAMTS13 deficiency is not a reason to withhold apheresis therapy. TPE with plasma-based fluid replacement has decreased the mortality from over 90% to between 10% and 20% (ASFA Category I).[102] If TPE is not readily available, infusion of plasma should be initiated (40 mL/kg or as tolerance allows) until apheresis therapy can be arranged. In conjunction with TPE, high-dose steroid therapy is often recommended, but no definitive trials to prove steroid efficacy have been performed.[102] Relapses are common, particularly in patients presenting with severe ADAMTS13 deficiency and an inhibitor. The role for rituximab to accelerate clinical resolution of symptoms and delay recurrences in acquired cases was shown in a Phase II trial.[108,109] Congenital deficiency of the metalloprotease ADAMTS13 is a rare autosomal recessive condition where prophylactic plasma infusion may be useful in disease management.

HUS is a TMA in which the renal vasculature thrombosis predominates, although other organ systems (such as brain and gastrointestinal tract) may also be affected. HUS is broadly classified as typical and atypical. Typical HUS is most appropriately referred to as STEC-HUS and generally related to Shiga-toxin-producing *Escherichia coli*. There is often a history of painful diarrhea in these patients; patients may present in epidemics, and markers for toxigenic *E. coli* or *Shigella* should be sought. Care of typical HUS is generally supportive.[105] The alternative form of HUS is designated atypical HUS. Up to 60% of patients with aHUS have inherited or acquired abnormalities affecting the components of the complement pathway (Factor H, Factor I, CD46, Factor B, C3, or thrombomodulin). There has been recognition that excessive activation of the alternative complement pathway underlies the pathogenesis of aHUS, and data has supported the efficacy of therapy aimed at inhibition of complement Factor C5. Thus, eculizumab, a humanized C5 monoclonal antibody (Soliris, Alexion, Cheshire, CT) is the preferred therapy over TPE for the long-term management of aHUS.[102,108,110]

Disorders of Fibrinolysis

Primary disorders of fibrinolysis are rare and hard to differentiate from DIC. Most fibrinolytic states are secondary to strong procoagulant stimuli. Antifibrinolytic therapy (with either EACA or tranexamic acid) has been reported to be successful in the treatment of surgical settings where bleeding is attributable to activation of the fibrinolytic mechanism, such as cardiopulmonary bypass procedures, liver transplantation, and massive trauma. However, the use of systemic antifibrinolytic therapy in other clinical settings may require a hematology consultation, because blockade of the fibrinolytic system can be associated with pathologic thrombosis.[22]

The therapeutic administration of the plasminogen activators such as recombinant tPA has grown increasingly important in the treatment of thrombotic disease. These agents may be used locally (ie, infused via angiographic control directly into the thrombosed area) or systemically (ie, infused via the peripheral vein). Successful results have been reported in coronary disease, cerebral disease, thromboembolic stroke, and peripheral arterial disease, as well as in pulmonary embolism and deep vein thrombosis. Contraindications to thrombolytic therapy include recent cranial trauma or known intracranial lesions and recent major surgery. Laboratory monitoring is not precise, and treatment regimens are standardized for each agent. The lytic state can be monitored by periodic assay of fibrinogen concentration, TT, or potentially viscoelastic testing. Discontinuation of the drug and repletion of fibrinogen with Cryoprecipitated AHF are useful if a patient develops uncontrolled bleeding while receiving thrombolytic agents. Inhibitors of fibrinolysis should be used with extreme caution in this setting.[64]

References

1. Fogarty PF, Kessler CM. Hemophilia A and B. In: Kitchens CS, Kessler CM, Konkle BA, eds. Consultative hemostasis and thrombosis. 3rd ed. Philadelphia: Elsevier Saunders, 2013:45-59.
2. Hoffman M, Cichon LJ. Practical coagulation for the blood banker. Transfusion 2013;53:1594-602.
3. Newman PJ, Newman DK. Platelets and the vessel wall. In: Orkin SH, Nathan DG, Ginsberg D, et al, eds. Nathan and Oski's hematology of infancy and childhood. 7th ed. Philadelphia: Saunders Elsevier, 2009:1379-98.
4. Furie B, Furie BC. In vivo thrombus formation. J Thromb Haemost 2007;5(Suppl 1):12-17.
5. Heit JA. Thrombophilia: Common questions on laboratory assessment and management. Hematol Am Soc Hematol Educ Program 2007:127-35.
6. Hajjar KA. The molelular basis of fibrinolysis. In: Orkin SH, Nathan DG, Ginsberg D, et al, eds. Nathan and Oski's hematology of infancy and childhood. 7th ed. Philadelphia: Saunders Elsevier, 2009:1425-48.
7. Brass L. Understanding and evaluating platelet function. Hematol Am Soc Hematol Educ Program 2010:387-96.
8. Kessler CM. A systematic approach to the bleeding patient: Correlation of clinical symptoms and signs with laboratory testing. In: Kitchens CS, Kessler CM, Konkle

BA, eds. Consultative hemostasis and thrombosis. 3rd ed. Philadelphia: Elsevier Saunders, 2013:16-32.
9. Favaloro EJ. Clinical utility of the PFA-100. Semin Thromb Hemost 2008;34:709-33.
10. Lisman T, Porte RJ. Rebalanced hemostasis in patients with liver disease: Evidence and clinical consequences. Blood 2010;116:878-85.
11. Zapotocka E, Curtin JA, Blanchette VS. Managing hemophilia in children and adolescents. In: Blanchette VS, Brandão LR, Breakey VR, Revel-Vilk S, eds. SickKids handbook of pediatric thrombosis and hemostasis. 2nd ed. Basel: Karger, 2017:71-96.
12. Peyvandi F, Menegatti M. Treatment of rare factor deficiencies in 2016. Hematol Am Soc Hematol Educ Program 2016:663-9.
13. Ferraris VA, Brown JR, Despotis GJ, et al. 2011 update to the Society of Thoracic Surgeons and the Society of Cardiovascular Anesthesiologists blood conservation clinical practice guidelines. Ann Thorac Surg 2011;91:944-82.
14. DeLoughery TG. Logistics of massive transfusions. Hematol Am Soc Hematol Educ Program 2010:470-3.
15. Bolliger D, Seeberger MD, Tanaka KA. Principles and practice of thromboelastography in clinical coagulation management and transfusion practice. Transfus Med Rev 2012;26:1-13.
16. Abeysundara L, Mallett SV, Clevenger B. Point-of-care testing in liver disease and liver surgery. Semin Thromb Hemost 2017;43:407-15.
17. Bochsen L, Wiinberg B, Kjelgaard-Hansen M, et al. Evaluation of the TEG platelet mapping assay in blood donors. Thromb J 2007;5:3.
18. Oliver WC. Anticoagulation and coagulation management for ECMO. Semin Cardiothorac Vasc Anesth 2009;13:154-75.
19. Afshari A, Wikkelso A, Brok J, et al. Thrombelastography (TEG) or thromboelastometry (ROTEM) to monitor hae-

motherapy versus usual care in patients with massive transfusion. Cochrane Database Syst Rev 2011;(3):CD007871.
20. Stravitz RT. Potential applications of thromboelastography in patients with acute and chronic liver disease. Gastroenterol Hepatol (N Y) 2012;8:513-20.
21. Coakley M, Reddy K, Mackie I, Mallett S. Transfusion triggers in orthotopic liver transplantation: A comparison of the thromboelastometry analyzer, the thromboelastogram, and conventional coagulation tests. J Cardiothorac Vasc Anesth 2006;20:548-53.
22. Hunt BJ. Bleeding and coagulopathies in critical care. N Engl J Med 2014;370:847-59.
23. British Committee for Haematology. Blood transfusion: Guidelines for the use of platelet transfusion. Br J Haematol 2003;122:10-23.
24. Kaufman RM, Djulbegovic B, Gernsheimer T, et al. Platelet transfusion: A clinical practice guideline from the AABB. Ann Intern Med 2015;162:205-13.
25. Slichter SJ. Evidence-based platelet transfusion guidelines. Hematol Am Soc Hematol Educ Program 2007:172-8.
26. Chakrabarti S, Varma S, Singh S, Kumari S. Low dose bolus aminocaproic acid: An alternative to platelet transfusion in thrombocytopenia? Eur J Haematol 1998;60:313-14.
27. Andrews J, Winkler AM. Challenges with navigating the precarious hemostatic balance during extracorporial life support: Implications for coagulation and transfusion management. Transfus Med Rev 2016;30:223-9.
28. Neunert C, Lim W, Crowther M, et al. The American Society of Hematology 2011 evidence-based practice guideline for immune thrombocytopenia. Blood 2011;117:4190-207.
29. Goel R, Ness PM, Takemoto CM, et al. Platelet transfusions in platelet consumptive disorders are associated with arterial thrombosis and in-hospital mortality. Blood 2015;125:1470-6.
30. Onwuemene O, Arepally GM. Heparin-induced thrombocytopenia: Research and clinical updates. Hematol Am Soc Hematol Educ Program 2016:262-8.

31. Swisher KK, Terrell DR, Vesely SK, et al. Clinical outcomes after platelet transfusions in patients with thrombotic thrombocytopenic purpura. Transfusion 2009; 49:873-87.
32. Jobe S, Di Paola J. Congenital and acquired disorders of platelet function and number. In: Kitchens CS, Kessler CM, Konkle BA, eds. Consultative hemostasis and thrombosis. 3rd ed. Philadelphia: Elsevier Saunders, 2013:132-49.
33. Bolton-Maggs PH, Chalmers EA, Collins PW, et al. A review of inherited platelet disorders with guidelines for their management on behalf of the UKHCDO. Br J Haematol 2006;135:603-33.
34. Chew DP, Moliterno DJ. A critical appraisal of platelet glycoprotein IIb/IIIa inhibition. J Am Coll Cardiol 2000; 36:2028-35.
35. Becker RC. Hemostatic aspects of cardiovascular medicine. In: Kitchens CS, Alving BM, Kitchens CS, eds. Consultative hemostasis and thrombosis. 2nd ed. Philadelphia: Saunders Elsevier, 2007:339-69.
36. Curtis BR, Divgi A, Garritty M, Aster RH. Delayed thrombocytopenia after treatment with abciximab: A distinct clinical entity associated with the immune response to the drug. J Thromb Haemost 2004;2:985-92.
37. Nichols WL, Hultin MB, James AH, et al. von Willebrand disease (VWD): Evidence-based diagnosis and management guidelines, the National Heart, Lung, and Blood Institute (NHLBI) Expert Panel report (USA). Haemophilia 2008;14:171-232.
38. Leebeek FWG, Eikenboom JCJ. von Willebrand's disease. N Engl J Med 2017;376:701-2.
39. Breakey VR, Carcao M. von Willebrand disease in children. In: Blanchette VS, Brandão LR, Breakey VR, Revel-Vilk S, eds. SickKids handbook of pediatric thrombosis and hemostasis. 2nd ed. Basel: Karger, 2017:97-112.
40. Federici AB, Budde U, Castaman G, et al. Current diagnostic and therapeutic approaches to patients with acquired

von Willebrand syndrome: A 2013 update. Semin Thromb Hemost 2013;39:191-201.
41. Bolan CD, Klein HG. Blood component and pharmacologic therapy for hemostatic disorders. In: Kitchens CS, Kessler CM, Konkle BA, eds. Consultative hemostasis and thrombosis. 3rd ed. Philadelphia: Elsevier Saunders, 2013:496-525.
42. Serrano K, Scammell K, Weiss S, et al. Plasma and cryoprecipitate manufactured from whole blood held overnight at room temperature meet quality standards. Transfusion 2010;50:344-53.
43. Mannucci PM. Treatment of von Willebrand's disease. N Engl J Med 2004;351:683-94.
44. Peyvandi F, Mannucci PM, Garagiola I, et al. A randomized trial of Factor VIII and neutralizing antibodies in hemophilia A. N Engl J Med 2016;374:2054-64.
45. Batorova A, Martinowitz U. Continuous infusion of coagulation factors: Current opinion. Curr Opin Hematol 2006;13:308-15.
46. Casana P, Martinez F, Haya S, et al. New mutations in exon 28 of the von Willebrand factor gene detected in patients with different types of von Willebrand's disease. Haematologica 2001;86:414-19.
47. Hay CR, Brown S, Collins PW, et al. The diagnosis and management of factor VIII and IX inhibitors: A guideline from the United Kingdom Haemophilia Centre Doctors Organisation. Br J Haematol 2006;133:591-605.
48. Mariani G, Herrmann FH, Schulman S, et al. Thrombosis in inherited factor VII deficiency. J Thromb Haemost 2003;1:2153-8.
49. Leissinger C, Gringeri A, Antmen B, et al. Anti-inhibitor coagulant complex prophylaxis in hemophilia with inhibitors. N Engl J Med 2011;365:1684-92.
50. Levi M, Levy JH, Andersen HF, Truloff D. Safety of recombinant activated factor VII in randomized clinical trials. N Engl J Med 2010;363:1791-800.

51. Kruse-Jarres R, St-Louis J, Greist A, et al. Efficacy and safety of OBI-1, an antihaemophilic factor VIII (recombinant), porcine sequence, in subjects with acquired haemophilia A. Haemophilia 2015;21:162-70.
52. Tarantino MD, Cuker A, Hardesty B, et al. Recombinant porcine sequence factor VIII (rpFVIII) for acquired haemophilia A: Practical clinical experience of its use in seven patients. Haemophilia 2017;23:25-32.
53. Kempton CL, White GC. How we treat a hemophilia A patient with a factor VIII inhibitor. Blood 2009;113:11-17.
54. Xavier F, Revel-Vilk S, Blanchette VS. Rare congenital factor deficiencies in childhood. In: Blanchette VS, Brandão LR, Breakey VR, Revel-Vilk S, eds. SickKids handbook of pediatric thrombosis and hemostasis. 2nd ed. Basel: Karger, 2017:113-31.
55. Austin SK, Brindley C, Kavakli K, et al. Pharmacokinetics of a high-purity plasma-derived factor X concentrate in subjects with moderate or severe hereditary factor X deficiency. Haemophilia 2016;22:426-32.
56. Scott E, Puca K, Heraly J, et al. Evaluation and comparison of coagulation factor activity in fresh-frozen plasma and 24-hour plasma at thaw and after 120 hours of 1 to 6 degrees C storage. Transfusion 2009;49:1584-91.
57. Yazer MH, Cortese-Hassett A, Triulzi DJ. Coagulation factor levels in plasma frozen within 24 hours of phlebotomy over 5 days of storage at 1 to 6 degrees C. Transfusion 2008;48:2525-30.
58. Inbal A, Oldenburg J, Carcao M, et al. Recombinant factor XIII: A safe and novel treatment for congenital factor XIII deficiency. Blood 2012;119:5111-17.
59. Levy JH, Welsby I, Goodnough LT. Fibrinogen as a therapeutic target for bleeding: A review of critical levels and replacement therapy. Transfusion 2014;54:1389-405.
60. Acharya SS, Dimichele DM. Rare inherited disorders of fibrinogen. Haemophilia 2008;14:1151-8.

61. Favier R, Aoki N, de Moerloose P. Congenital alpha(2)-plasmin inhibitor deficiencies: A review. Br J Haematol 2001;114:4-10.
62. Eichinger S. Reversing vitamin K antagonists: Making the old new again. Hematol Am Soc Hematol Educ Program 2016:605-11.
63. Schulman S, Beyth RJ, Kearon C, Levine MN. Hemorrhagic complications of anticoagulant and thrombolytic treatment: American College of Chest Physicians Evidence-Based Clinical Practice Guidelines (8th Edition). Chest 2008;133:257S-98S.
64. Makris M, van Veen JJ, Tait CR, et al. Guideline on the management of bleeding in patients on antithrombotic agents. Br J Haematol 2013;160:35-46.
65. Schulman S, Bijsterveld NR. Anticoagulants and their reversal. Transfus Med Rev 2007;21:37-48.
66. Di Nisio M, Middeldorp S, Büller HR. Direct thrombin inhibitors. N Engl J Med 2005;353:1028-40.
67. Cuker A, Siegal DM, Crowther MA, Garcia DA. Laboratory measurement of the anticoagulant activity of the non-vitamin K oral anticoagulants. J Am Coll Cardiol 2014; 64:1128-39.
68. Pollack CV Jr, Reilly PA, Eikelboom J, et al. Idarucizumab for dabigatran reversal. N Engl J Med 2015;373:511-20.
69. Shih AW, Crowther MA. Reversal of direct oral anticoagulants: A practical approach. Hematol Am Soc Hematol Educ Program 2016:612-19.
70. Douketis JD. Pharmacologic properties of the new oral anticoagulants: A clinician-oriented review with a focus on perioperative management. Curr Pharm Des 2010;16:3436-41.
71. Sarode R, Milling TJ Jr, Refaai MA, et al. Efficacy and safety of a 4-factor prothrombin complex concentrate in patients on vitamin K antagonists presenting with major bleeding: A randomized, plasma-controlled, phase IIIb study. Circulation 2013;128:1234-43.

72. Connolly SJ, Milling TJ Jr, Eikelboom JW, et al. Andexanet alfa for acute major bleeding associated with factor xa inhibitors. N Engl J Med 2016;375:1131-41.
73. Ansell JE, Bakhru SH, Laulicht BE, et al. Single-dose ciraparantag safely and completely reverses anticoagulant effects of edoxaban. Thromb Haemost 2017;117:238-45.
74. Eikelboom JW, Hirsh J, Spencer FA, et al. Antiplatelet drugs: Antithrombotic therapy and prevention of thrombosis. 9th ed: American College of Chest Physicians evidence-based clinical practice guidelines. Chest 2012;141(2 Suppl):e89S-e119S.
75. Brilinta package insert. London, UK: AstraZeneca, 2014. [Available at https://www.accessdata.fda.gov/drugsatfda_docs/label/2015/022433s017lbl.pdf (accessed July 17, 2017).]
76. Baharoglu MI, Cordonnier C, Al-Shahi SR, et al. Platelet transfusion versus standard care after acute stroke due to spontaneous cerebral haemorrhage associated with antiplatelet therapy (PATCH): A randomised, open-label, phase 3 trial. Lancet 2016;387:2605-13.
77. Messmore HL Jr, Jeske WP, Wehrmacher W, et al. Antiplatelet agents: Current drugs and future trends. Hematol Oncol Clin North Am 2005;19:87-117, vi.
78. Tripodi A, Mannucci PM. The coagulopathy of chronic liver disease. N Engl J Med 2011;365:147-56.
79. Segal JB, Dzik WH. Paucity of studies to support that abnormal coagulation test results predict bleeding in the setting of invasive procedures: An evidence-based review. Transfusion 2005;45:1413-25.
80. Youssef WI, Salazar F, Dasarathy S, et al. Role of fresh frozen plasma infusion in correction of coagulopathy of chronic liver disease: A dual phase study. Am J Gastroenterol 2003;98:1391-4.
81. Lisman T, Porte RJ. Understanding and managing the coagulopathy of liver disease. In: Kitchens CS, Kessler CM, Konkle BA, eds. Consultative hemostasis and throm-

bosis. 3rd ed. Philadelphia: Elsevier Saunders, 2013:688-97.
82. De Pietri L, Bianchini M, Montalti R, et al. Thrombelastography-guided blood product use before invasive procedures in cirrhosis with severe coagulopathy: A randomized, controlled trial. Hepatology 2016;63:566-73.
83. Logan AC, Goodnough LT. Recombinant factor VIIa: An assessment of evidence regarding its efficacy and safety in the off-label setting. Hematol Am Soc Hematol Educ Program 2010:153-9.
84. Levi M. Disseminated intravascular coagulation. Crit Care Med 2007;35:2191-5.
85. Levi M, Toh CH, Thachil J, Watson HG. Guidelines for the diagnosis and management of disseminated intravascular coagulation. British Committee for Standards in Haematology. Br J Haematol 2009;145:24-33.
86. White NJ. Mechanisms of trauma-induced coagulopathy. Hematol Am Soc Hematol Educ Program 2013:660-3.
87. Holcomb JB, Pati S. Optimal trauma resuscitation with plasma as the primary resuscitative fluid: The surgeon's perspective. Hematol Am Soc Hematol Educ Program 2013:656-9.
88. Holcomb JB. Optimal use of blood products in severely injured trauma patients. Hematol Am Soc Hematol Educ Program 2010:465-9.
89. Chandler WL, Ferrell C, Trimble S, Moody S. Development of a rapid emergency hemorrhage panel. Transfusion 2010;50:2547-52.
90. Kashuk JL, Moore EE, Wohlauer M, et al. Initial experiences with point-of-care rapid thrombelastography for management of life-threatening postinjury coagulopathy. Transfusion 2012;52:23-33.
91. Stainsby D, MacLennan S, Thomas D, et al. Guidelines on the management of massive blood loss. Br J Haematol 2006;135:634-41.

92. Roberts I, Shakur H, Afolabi A, et al. The importance of early treatment with tranexamic acid in bleeding trauma patients: An exploratory analysis of the CRASH-2 randomised controlled trial. Lancet 2011;377:1096-101, 1101.e1-2.
93. Gruen RL, Mitra B. Tranexamic acid for trauma. Lancet 2011;377:1052-4.
94. Hess JR. Resuscitation of trauma-induced coagulopathy. Hematol Am Soc Hematol Educ Program 2013:664-7.
95. Etchill EW, Myers SP, McDaniel LM, et al. Should all massively transfused patients be treated equally? An analysis of massive transfusion ratios in the nontrauma setting. Crit Care Med 2017;45:1311-16.
96. Bauer KA. Duration of anticoagulation: Applying the guidelines and beyond. Hematol Am Soc Hematol Educ Program 2010:210-15.
97. Guyatt GH, Akl EA, Crowther M, et al. Executive summary: Antithrombotic therapy and prevention of thrombosis, 9th ed: American College of Chest Physicians evidence-based clinical practice guidelines. Chest 2012; 141:7S-47S.
98. Heit JA. Thrombophilia: Clinical and laboratory assessment and management. In: Kitchens CS, Kessler CM, Konkle BA, eds. Consultative hemostasis and thrombosis. 3rd ed. Philadelphia: Elsevier Saunders, 2013:205-39.
99. Gosselin R, Grant RP, Adcock DM. Comparison of the effect of the anti-Xa direct oral anticoagulants apixaban, edoxaban, and rivaroxaban on coagulation assays. Int J Lab Hematol 2016;38:505-13.
100. Goldenberg NA, Manco-Johnson MJ. Protein C deficiency. Haemophilia 2008;14:1214-21.
101. Lim W. Antiphospholipid syndrome. Hematol Am Soc Hematol Educ Program 2013:675-80.
102. Schwartz J, Padmanabhan A, Aqui N, et al. Guidelines on the use of therapeutic apheresis in clinical practice—evidence-based approach from the Writing Committee of

the American Society for Apheresis: The seventh special issue. J Clin Apher 2016;31:149-62.
103. Raflores MB, Kaplan RB, Spero JA. Pre-operative management of a patient with hypoprothrombinemia-lupus anticoagulant syndrome. Thromb Haemost 2007;98:248-50.
104. Padmanabhan A, Jones CG, Pechauer SM, et al. IVIg for treatment of severe refractory heparin-induced thrombocytopenia. Chest 2017 Apr 17. pii: S0012-3692(17)30724-9. doi: 10.1016/j.chest.2017.03.050. [Epub ahead of print.]
105. George JN, Nester CM. Syndromes of thrombotic microangiopathy. N Engl J Med 2014;371:654-66.
106. Masias C, Vasu S, Cataland SR. None of the above: Thrombotic microangiopathy beyond TTP and HUS. Blood 2017;129:2857-63.
107. Joly BS, Coppo P, Veyradier A. Thrombotic thrombocytopenic purpura. Blood 2017;129:2836-46.
108. Scully M, Goodship T. How I treat thrombotic thrombocytopenic purpura and atypical haemolytic uraemic syndrome. Br J Haematol 2014;164:759-66.
109. Scully M, McDonald V, Cavenagh J, et al. A phase 2 study of the safety and efficacy of rituximab with plasma exchange in acute acquired thrombotic thrombocytopenic purpura. Blood 2011;118:1746-53.
110. Legendre CM, Licht C, Muus P, et al. Terminal complement inhibitor eculizumab in atypical hemolytic-uremic syndrome. N Engl J Med 2013;368:2169-81.

TRANSFUSION PRACTICES

Surgical Blood Ordering Practices

Type and Screen

A type and screen (T/S) order involves typing the patient's red cells for ABO and Rh type, and screening the patient's serum for clinically significant red cell alloantibodies. These are antibodies that are capable of causing red cell destruction after transfusion of incompatible red cells. A T/S order is recommended for surgical procedures with minimal blood loss, which are defined as procedures requiring no blood transfusion in 90% of cases. When the antibody screen is negative, no clinically significant red cell antibodies are identified. When the screen is positive, clinically significant antibodies may be present. When this happens, the blood bank will proceed with antibody identification and reserve antigen-negative units for the patient.[1]

Type and Crossmatch

A type and crossmatch (T/C) is the same as a T/S except that blood is selected and reserved for the patient. A T/C is ordered when red cell transfusion is anticipated. For surgical procedures, a T/C is ordered for procedures that involve blood loss and require transfusion in 90% of cases based on the maximum surgical blood order schedule (MSBOS). (See Chapter 5: Patient Blood Management.)

If the antibody screen is negative and no clinically significant red cell antibodies are identified, an electronic crossmatch or a rapid serologic crossmatch can be performed (see Fig 1). The manual rapid crossmatch serves only to confirm ABO compatibility between the patient and the unit (see Table 10). In many hospitals, the rapid crossmatch has been replaced with an electronic crossmatch, in which ABO and Rh compatibility are confirmed and units are crossmatched using computer software.[1,2] For patients with a negative antibody screen, ABO-specific crossmatched blood can be available in 10 to 15 minutes.

If the patient's serum contains clinically significant red cell antibodies, an antiglobulin crossmatch is mandatory[1] and will require an additional 30 to 60 minutes to complete before units can be released for transfusion. To prevent unexpected delays, the blood bank may frequently locate and crossmatch units to ensure that blood will be available during surgery within the 10- to 15-minute time frame.

Delays may occur when patients who are to undergo surgery are admitted to the hospital on the day of surgery, because the blood bank may not have sufficient time to identify a clinically significant antibody and then find crossmatch-compatible units. This process takes a minimum of 90 minutes to complete for patients with a simple antibody, and it can take hours to days in complicated cases. To prevent this delay, patients should have blood specimens drawn for compatibility testing well in advance of the need for blood, particularly those patients with a history of blood exposure from pregnancy or transfusion.

Some programs have established an extended preoperative T/S policy for elective surgery patients with a negative antibody screen and no history of either transfusion or pregnancy within the preceding 3 months. In these patients, samples can be drawn up to 1 month ahead of the time of surgery.[3] This is not true for patients with a positive screen or a history of a clinically significant alloantibody. In these patients, a current blood specimen is required to crossmatch units for surgery.[2] Preoperative blood ordering schedules are used to predict surgical blood needs and

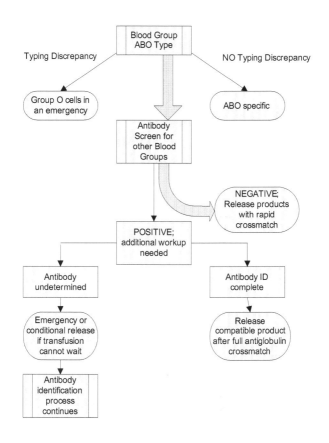

Figure 1. Sample processing for ABO type, antibody screen, and crossmatch *[Courtesy Roberta Arney, MT(ASCP)SBB]*.

Table 10. ABO Compatibility

Patient ABO Blood Group			Blood Compatibility	
Red Cell Antigens	**Plasma Antibodies**	**ABO Type**	**RBCs**	**Plasma**
A	Anti-B	A	A, O	A, AB
B	Anti-A	B	B, O	B, AB
A and B	None	AB	A, B, AB, O	AB
None	Anti-A, -B	O	O	A, B, AB, O

RBCs = Red Blood Cells.

efficiently allocate blood on the day of surgery. (See Chapter 5: Patient Blood Management.)

Urgent Transfusion

Urgent transfusion refers to the administration of blood components [typically Red Blood Cell (RBC) units] before the completion of standard pretransfusion testing, when a delay in transfusion may imperil the patient. Further information on the risks and medical management of bleeding emergencies can be found in Chapter 5 (Patient Blood Management) and Chapter 6 (Blood Component Resuscitation in Trauma and Massive Bleeding).

If transfusion is necessary before completion of pretransfusion testing, group O RBCs should be used. If the ABO type is known, the patient can receive type-specific RBCs. Whenever possible, D-negative RBCs should be used for females of childbearing potential and children to avoid the possibility of sensitization to the D antigen. Patients requiring plasma should receive type-specific plasma if an ABO type is known. In patients without an ABO type on file, group AB or A plasma may be provided.[4]

Either before or after the uncrossmatched blood is issued, the patient's physician must sign a statement indicating the nature of the emergency. If the patient's screen for unexpected red cell antibodies is negative, the transfusion of uncrossmatched RBCs carries a very low risk of incompatibility.[5,6] However, this safety margin depends on the correct identification of the patient, the pretransfusion blood sample, and the blood components to be infused.

Hematopoietic Progenitor Cell Transplantation

Hematopoietic progenitor cells (HPCs) are primitive cells capable of self-renewal and differentiation into committed hematopoietic cells.[7] Sources of HPCs include marrow (HPC, Marrow), peripheral blood (HPC, Apheresis), and umbilical cord blood (HPC, Cord Blood). The choice of stem cell source is influenced by the patient's disease, the HLA-best-matched donor, donor availability, and donor safety. HPCs may be obtained from the patient (autologous) or a related or unrelated donor (allogeneic). Allogeneic HPCs are used for treatment of leukemia, marrow failure, congenital immunodeficiency syndromes, some hemoglobinopathies, and inborn errors of metabolism. Autologous HPC therapy is used as rescue therapy following myeloablative high-dose chemotherapy/radiation. Diseases often treated by autologous HPC transplantation include plasma cell dyscrasias, lymphoma, pediatric cancers, and autoimmune disorders.[7]

Patients undergoing HPC transplantation require RBC and platelet support during the period of marrow aplasia. In autologous and allogeneic transplantation of HPC, Apheresis, this period may extend for 2 to 3 weeks depending on the HPC transplant dose, ABO compatibility, and infection. In contrast, cord blood transplant recipients often require extended transfusion support because of delayed marrow engraftment. For RBC transfusions, it is common practice to maintain a hemoglobin level greater than 8 to 9 g/dL in outpatients. In the inpatient setting, recent studies have shown that a lower trigger (hemoglobin >7 g/dL) is safe in hospitalized neutropenic patients.[8,9] Transfusion guidelines for platelet transfusions are similar to those for oncology patients undergoing chemotherapy, with prophylactic platelet transfusion administered at platelet counts below 10,000/mL.[10,11]

All HPC transplantation recipients require T-cell-inactivated (irradiated or pathogen-reduced) blood components (RBCs and platelets) to prevent graft-vs-host disease (GVHD). In addition, RBCs and platelets should be leukocyte reduced to prevent HLA alloimmunization and potential transfusion-transmitted cytomegalovirus (CMV). (See Chapter 1: Blood Components; Chapter 7: Adverse Effects of Blood Transfusion.) Patients who have undergone an ABO-mismatched, allogeneic HPC transplantation require additional blood selection criteria. Although primitive HPCs lack ABO antigens, ABO incompatibility between donor and recipient can lead to delayed RBC engraftment or late hemolysis of donor RBCs because of residual anti-A and/or anti-B in the recipient.[12] As a consequence, blood components are selected that are compatible with the donor and the recipient (see Table 11).

Solid Organ Transplantation

The transplantation of solid organs such as the kidney, heart, lung, small bowel, and liver can also present challenges for transfusion therapy. The transplant procedure and perioperative

Table 11. Transfusion Support for Patients Undergoing ABO-Mismatched Allogeneic HPC Transplantation

Recipient	Donor	Mismatch Type	Preparative Regimen Through Transplantation (while recipient antibodies are detected)				Recipient Antibodies No Longer Detected
			RBCs	Platelets*	Plasma		All Components
A	O	Minor	O	A	A		Donor
B	O	Minor	O	B	B		Donor
AB	O	Minor	O	AB	AB		Donor
AB	A	Minor	A	AB	AB		Donor
AB	B	Minor	B	AB	AB		Donor
O	A	Major	O	A	A		Donor
O	B	Major	O	B	B		Donor
O	AB	Major	O	AB	AB		Donor

(Continued)

Table 11. Transfusion Support for Patients Undergoing ABO-Mismatched Allogeneic HPC Transplantation (Continued)

Recipient	Donor	Mismatch Type	Preparative Regimen Through Transplantation (while recipient antibodies are detected)				Recipient Antibodies No Longer Detected
			RBCs	Platelets*	Plasma		All Components
A	AB	Major	A	AB	AB		Donor
B	AB	Major	B	AB	AB		Donor
A	B	Minor and major	O	AB	AB		Donor
B	A	Minor and major	O	AB	AB		Donor

All cellular components should be irradiated and leukocyte reduced.

*Due to the short shelf life and limited availability of group AB platelets, it may not always be possible to provide fully matched ABO platelet products as recommended in the table. Therefore, blood banks and transfusion services may consider providing ABO-mismatched platelets that have been volume reduced to diminish their plasma content.

HPC = hematopoietic progenitor cell; RBCs = Red Blood Cells.

period may be associated with substantial bleeding and massive transfusion. Solid organ transplant surgeries, except kidney, typically require both RBC and plasma transfusion. Liver patients are at increased risk for citrate-induced hypocalcemia from liver dysfunction and rapid transfusion.[13] Liver transplant patients often have complex preoperative coagulopathies that may be compounded during the anhepatic phase of surgery to yield profound hemostatic derangements.

In general, transplanted organs are ABO compatible with the recipient. Transplantation of organs across major ABO barriers can result in acute rejection. Criteria and protocols for transplanting across ABO types in solid organ transplantation in children and adults have been published with acceptable long-term graft survival.[14-16] Neonates are considered good candidates for ABO-incompatible transplantation because of low or absent ABO antibodies.[14,16] Transplantation of major-ABO-incompatible kidneys and hearts often requires preoperative B-cell depletion and plasma exchange to decrease ABO antibody titers, combined with aggressive immunosuppression after transplantation.[14,15] (See Chapter 8: Therapeutic Apheresis.) Plasma components (plasma and platelets) should be selected that are compatible with both the patient's red cells and the transplanted organ. Minor ABO incompatibility is not as great a concern as major ABO incompatibility for intraoperative support; however, it can be associated with significant hemolytic anemia 10 to 21 days after surgery because of ABO (or other red cell) antibody production by passenger graft lymphocytes in the transplanted organ.[12]

GVHD is not commonly seen after solid organ transplantation and is usually associated with passenger lymphocytes in donor organs. Because cases of transfusion-associated GVHD (TA-GVHD) have occurred only rarely in this setting, the use of T-cell-inactivated blood components for solid organ recipients is not routinely required. (See Chapter 7: Adverse Effects of Blood Transfusion.)

Obstetric Transfusion Practices

Hemolytic Disease of the Fetus and Newborn

Fetal red cells can express red cell antigens inherited from the father that may be absent in the mother. Because fetomaternal hemorrhages occur in nearly all pregnancies, a small percentage of mothers (0.06%-0.24%) make antibodies against these paternally derived red cell antigens.[17] These maternal red cell alloantibodies can lead to hemolytic disease of the fetus and newborn (HDFN), in which maternal immunoglobulin G (IgG) antibodies are transported across the placenta and opsonize fetal red cells, leading to extravascular hemolysis of fetal red cells within the spleen. HDFN can vary in severity from IgG sensitization of fetal red cells without apparent hemolysis to hydropic death in utero caused by severe anemia. IgM antibodies (eg, anti-I, anti-Lea, and anti-P1) do not cause HDFN because, unlike IgG, they cannot cross the placenta.

The most common cause of clinically significant HDFN is antibody to the RhD antigen. The incidence of Rh HDFN has declined from 13% to 0.04%,[18] primarily as a result of the use of Rh Immune Globulin (RhIG). The administration of this hyperimmune globulin prevents D immunization in pregnant women who are D negative. ABO incompatibility between mother and fetus can also lead to HDFN, although it is seldom clinically significant.[17] Many other blood group antigens, such as Kell, Duffy, and other Rh system antigens, can also cause maternal alloimmunization and HDFN. Antibodies against Kell (K1) antigen have been associated with severe reticulocytopenic HDFN and mild thrombocytopenia from hemolysis and suppression of fetal hematopoiesis.[19] As a consequence, some European countries prophylactically provide K1-negative RBCs to all K1-negative women of childbearing potential to prevent alloimmunization. The effectiveness of this strategy has been challenged in a recent study which has shown that transfusion accounts for only 3% of maternal alloimmunization: The vast majority of women (83%) are alloimmunized by a prior pregnancy.[20]

The goals of antibody screening in obstetric patients are the identification and monitoring of those females with blood group antibodies capable of causing HDFN, and the identification of D-negative females who should receive RhIG.[1,17] Testing at an early prenatal visit should include ABO and Rh typing, as well as an antibody screen designed to detect those red cell antibodies known to cause HDFN. If the initial antibody screen is negative, a repeat antibody screen at 28 to 30 weeks of gestation should be considered in D-negative females to detect early D alloimmunization.[17,18,21] A 300-µg dose of prophylactic RhIG is administered at this time to all D-negative females. In some countries, there are policies to target and limit RhIG prophylaxis to D-negative women based on molecular D typing of fetal cell-free DNA circulating in maternal plasma. In the Netherlands, the false-negative rate for fetal D typing (D-positive fetus typed as D negative) is 0.03%, whereas the false-negative rate for cord blood is 0.09%.[22] If fetal blood type is determined by using genetic testing, cautious interpretation may be necessary because of the complexity of the Rh loci, particularly among persons of African ancestry.[21,22]

After delivery, all nonalloimmunized D-negative mothers of D-positive infants must receive a second dose of at least 300 µg of RhIG within 72 hours of birth. A test should be performed to assess whether excessive fetomaternal hemorrhage has occurred, in order to determine whether additional RhIG must be administered to prevent D immunization.[17,18,21] (See Rh Immune Globulin in Chapter 2: Plasma Derivatives.)

Once it has been ascertained that a mother has become alloimmunized, the management of the pregnancy is guided by laboratory testing and ultrasound. When an antibody that is associated with HDFN is identified, an antibody titration is performed and repeated at regular intervals. If a "critical tube-titer" of anti-D of 16 or higher is reached, the risk of fetal hydrops after 18 to 20 weeks becomes significant, and further monitoring is indicated.[17,18,21] This can include amniocentesis, middle cerebral artery peak systolic velocity (MCA-PSV) Doppler, and direct fetal blood sampling.[23]

The predictive value of titers for alloantibodies other than anti-D is uncertain, but a rising titer (more than a fourfold or two-tube dilution increase) suggests that the fetus is at risk for HDFN and warrants more vigilant monitoring.[21] Caution is warranted when comparing and interpreting titers performed by different serologic methods. The risk of HDFN may be estimated by determining the father's red cell phenotype.[17] Alternatively, fetal blood type for non-D antigens can also be determined directly by DNA typing of fetal DNA in maternal plasma, amniotic fluid cells, or chorionic villi.[18,21]

Intrauterine Transfusion

Historically, pregnancies complicated by HDFN were monitored by serial measurements of amniotic fluid bilirubin via amniocentesis to assess the severity of hemolysis and detect possible hydrops. This has largely been replaced by MCA-PSV Doppler ultrasound, a highly accurate, noninvasive method for diagnosing and monitoring the severity of anemia, as well as the fetal response to transfusion therapy.[19,21]

When severe HDFN is suspected and the fetus cannot be delivered safely, more invasive procedures are necessary. Percutaneous umbilical blood sampling (PUBS) permits antenatal blood typing, precise monitoring of fetal hematocrit, and/or direct intravascular transfusion (IVT) of the fetus. However, the rate of fetal loss from a PUBS procedure is 1% to 2%, and the procedure is not performed unless necessary.[21] A severely affected fetus may receive blood either by IVT or, much less commonly, by intraperitoneal transfusion at periodic intervals until assessment of fetal viability indicates sufficient maturity for delivery.

Intrauterine transfusion is generally recommended when the fetal hematocrit decreases below 30%, but it is rarely feasible before 20 weeks of gestation. The volume transfused is determined according to the gestational age, estimated fetal blood volume, and technique to be used for transfusion. The transfusion is administered via cannulation of the umbilical vein under ultrasound guidance, and it generally achieves a 10% increase in hematocrit.[21,23,24] The goal of transfusion is a fetal hematocrit of 25% to 50%, but this endpoint should not exceed more than a fourfold increase over the pretransfusion hematocrit to avoid unfavorable viscosity changes in profoundly anemic fetuses. The hematocrit is expected to decline about 1% per day, and additional IVT procedures are performed to maintain a fetal hematocrit of 40% to 50%. This usually requires IVT every 2 weeks initially and tapering to every 3 to 4 weeks after suppression of erythropoiesis.[23] Transfusions are continued until the infant is viable for delivery.[21]

RBCs for transfusion should be crossmatch compatible with the mother's serum.[1,21,25] The units selected are typically group O, D-negative, hemoglobin-S-negative RBCs that lack the antigen corresponding to the maternal antibody. Fresh blood, usually less than 1 week old, is preferred to ensure maximum red cell viability and to avoid low pH, decreased red cell 2,3-diphosphoglycerate (2,3-DPG), and high plasma potassium levels. The hematocrit of the RBC unit should generally be 75% to 85% to decrease the risk of volume overload in the fetus. RBCs should be irradiated to prevent GVHD. To prevent transfusion-transmitted CMV, RBCs should be leukocyte reduced or CMV seronegative.[25] (See Chapter 1: Blood Components; Chapter 7: Adverse Effects of Blood Transfusion.)

Neonatal Transfusion Practices

Exchange Transfusion

Infants with HDFN and hyperbilirubinemia may require treatment with phototherapy, intravenous immune globulin (IVIG), or exchange transfusion. Exchange transfusion is usually reserved for severe hemolysis. Exchange transfusion corrects anemia and removes both antibody and potentially dangerous concentrations of bilirubin.

A 2-volume exchange will remove 85% of red cells, and lower bilirubin by 25% to 45%.[26] Reconstituted whole blood (ie, RBCs reconstituted with group AB plasma from a different donor) is most commonly used for exchange transfusion, with a final hematocrit of around 50% to 60%. The latter should result in a posttransfusion hemoglobin level of >12 g/dL.[27] A postexchange complete blood count (CBC) should be performed to monitor hematocrit and platelet count.

RBCs for exchange transfusion should be compatible with the mother's serum and ABO compatible with the infant. Blood less than 7 days old is usually used to ensure maximum red cell viability and to avoid decreased 2,3-DPG and high potassium levels. If fresh RBCs are unavailable, older units can be washed. As with intrauterine transfusion, RBC units should be hemoglobin S negative, leukocyte reduced (CMV safe), and irradiated to prevent TA-GVHD.[25]

Neonatal Thrombocytopenia

Approximately 1% of newborns are thrombocytopenic at birth.[28] Severe thrombocytopenia can be the consequence of congenital infections, congenital heart disease, sepsis and disseminated intravascular coagulation, chromosomal abnormalities, maternal immune thrombocytopenia (ITP), and neonatal alloimmune thrombocytopenia (NAIT). Both maternal ITP and NAIT are caused by the passive transfer of maternal antibodies that are reactive against the infant's platelets. NAIT occurs in approximately 1 in 1200 live births and is an important cause of isolated postnatal thrombocytopenia in an otherwise healthy term infant.[28,29]

Analogous to HDFN being a reaction against red cell antigens, NAIT is the result of maternal antibodies directed against platelet antigens on fetal platelets, particularly human platelet antigen (HPA)-1a (PlA1). Whereas maternal ITP typically runs a benign course in the infant, NAIT frequently affects the firstborn infant and can cause serious intracranial hemorrhage, even before delivery. This condition may be treated in utero by the administration of IVIG to the mother. Fetal blood sampling and direct IVT of compatible platelets is no longer recommended because of the high incidence (6%) of serious complications.[28]

It may also be necessary to transfuse platelets and IVIG after birth. Indications for transfusion include signs of bleeding and/or a platelet count <30,000/mL. Patients with platelet counts >30,000/mL and without bleeding can be managed with IVIG alone.[29]

For transfusion, leukocyte-reduced, ABO-compatible, whole-blood-derived platelets have been shown to be efficacious and are used as first-line treatment.[28,30] IVIG is often administered to prolong platelet survival and hasten patient recovery.[29,30] HPA-matched apheresis platelets may be obtained by plateletpheresis of the mother or through a rare donor registry. Maternal platelets must be washed to remove platelet alloantibody and be T-cell inactivated before transfusion.[29]

Routine Transfusion in Neonatal Patients

Two types of anemia develop in premature infants—iatrogenic and physiologic. In critically ill neonates, iatrogenic blood losses from repeated blood sampling required for laboratory monitoring can reach 5% of the total blood volume per day, and they are a major factor driving transfusion.[31] Physiologic anemia or anemia of prematurity develops a few weeks after birth as a result of decreased erythropoietin (EPO) production and responsiveness, reduced red cell life span, and hyporegenerative marrow.[31] Recombinant human EPO (rHuEPO) has not been shown to reduce transfusion needs or morbidity in sick neonates, while it increases the risk of retinopathy of prematurity.[31,32] In contrast, studies with darbepoetin, a long-acting EPO analogue, in low-birthweight infants suggest a decrease in transfusion requirements, improved cognitive outcomes, and no increase in retinopathy.[33]

The indications for transfusion in the neonate differ from those in the adult because of the infant's physiologic immaturity, small blood volume, and inability to tolerate procedure-related stress. RBC transfusion in very-low-birthweight infants may, in fact, increase the risk for intraventricular hemorrhage during the first week of life.[34]

The decision to transfuse must not be made on the basis of hemoglobin concentration alone, but rather on the basis of multiple factors, including calculated blood loss (generally 5% to 10% of total blood volume) over time, expected hemoglobin levels, reticulocyte count, and clinical status (eg, dyspnea, apnea, pallor, and poor weight gain).[31,32] Randomized controlled trials comparing lower vs higher hemoglobin threshold levels are conflicting, particularly with regard to the effect on long-term neurodevelopmental outcomes.[35-37]

Laboratory practices regarding RBC preparation can vary between institutions. Generally, RBC transfusions consist of an aliquot taken from a fresh blood unit. Even from older units, the amount of potassium infused in a small-volume transfusion (<10-15 mL/kg) is clinically insignificant if the blood is transfused over a 2-hour period at a steady rate.[31] The transfusion of 10 mL/kg of RBCs over a 2- to 3-hour period should raise the hemoglobin concentration by approximately 2 to 3 g/dL.[25,31]

To minimize donor exposures in an infant likely to require several transfusions, some institutions will assign a specific RBC unit to that infant. A sterile connecting device is used to withdraw sequential blood aliquots for small-volume transfusions from the same unit until its outdate.[38] This protocol is applicable only to those routine transfusions that can be given slowly (2 hours) by infusion pump, and not for massive or exchange transfusions.

For large-volume transfusion (≥ 20 mL/kg), RBCs that are either <7 days of age or washed are recommended to minimize potassium content.[31,39] RBCs in either citrate-phosphate-dextrose-adenine-1 or additive solutions can be used safely for transfusions.[31,32] The use of large-bore peripheral venous catheters, slower infusion rates, and frequent electrolyte monitoring may help avoid serious hypocalcemia and hyperkalemia.[39]

Infants less than 4 months old rarely produce antibodies to blood group antigens; therefore, standards for pretransfusion serologic testing of these patients are different from those for testing of older infants, children, and adults.[1] A pretransfusion ABO and Rh typing and an antibody screen must be performed. For neonates, maternal serum can be used for the antibody screening because any antibodies present in the infant are passively transferred from mother to infant during gestation.[17] If a clinically significant antibody is present in either maternal or fetal serum, RBC units lacking the corresponding antigen should be prepared for transfusion until the antibody is no longer identified in the infant's serum. If the initial antibody screen is negative, however, additional testing (eg, crossmatch) can be omitted, provided that 1) RBCs are group O or ABO-identical or -compatible with both the mother and child and 2) RBCs are either D negative or the same D antigen type as the infant. Repeat testing may be omitted for infants less than 4 months of age during any one hospital admission as long as they are receiving only group O cells.[1]

In general, the primary use of plasma is in the treatment of coagulation disorders. It is not recommended to treat hypovolemia only. Caution should be used in interpreting coagulation studies in polycythemic samples because of the excess citrate:plasma ratios in these samples.[27] As with adults, a dose of 10 to 15 mL/kg is recommended.[25,27] Plasma should be either group AB or ABO compatible with the recipient.

Platelet transfusion practices are variable and include establishing the platelet level at which prophylactic transfusions are given to sick premature infants.[25,27] In stable-term infants, bleeding is unlikely to occur at a platelet count of 20,000/µL. In sick infants, a platelet count >50,000/µL or platelet mass >400 fl/µL is recommended to decrease the risk of intraventricular hemorrhage.[33] Neonates on ECMO or undergoing surgery are transfused to maintain a platelet count >100,000/µL.[33] Platelets prepared for transfusion should be ABO identical or plasma compatible with the patient. A dose of 5 to 10 mL/kg is sufficient to increase the platelet count by 50,000 to 100,000/µL.[25,27]

T-cell inactivation is indicated for RBC and platelet transfusions in low-birthweight premature infants, patients undergoing exchange transfusion, patients with a congenital disorder of cellular immunity, or patients receiving directed donations from first-degree relatives to prevent GVHD. Although most cases of postnatal CMV infections are from maternal transmission through breast milk,[40] it is recommended that transfused RBCs and platelets be leukocyte reduced or CMV safe in neonates.

Granulocyte transfusions have been used in some institutions for septic and neutropenic patients. The efficacy of granulocyte transfusions vs granulocyte colony-stimulating factor in septic and neutropenic neonates is not fully established.[41] Granulocytes must be irradiated before transfusion regardless of patient age or underlying diagnosis. Because granulocytes cannot be leukocyte reduced, granulocytes should be CMV serocompatible with the recipient. (See Chapter 1: Blood Components.)

Pediatric Transfusion Practices

Transfusion in Older Infants and Children

The clinical decision to transfuse RBCs or other blood components to older infants and children is based on the same indications as those used for adults. Differences in blood volume, the ability to tolerate blood loss, and the normal hemoglobin and hematocrit levels for the age group in question are taken into consideration. Randomized studies have shown that stable, critically ill children can tolerate a hemoglobin level of 7 g/dL without an increase in morbidity or mortality.[42]

Sickle Cell Disease and Related Disorders

In certain chronic congenital anemias, RBC transfusions are used to suppress endogenous hemoglobin production. Children with thalassemia syndromes are given routine RBC transfusions to prevent tissue hypoxia and to suppress endogenous erythropoiesis so as to support more normal growth and development. Likewise, children with sickle cell disease who are at increased risk for a cerebrovascular accident, or who have undergone major splenic sequestration and are not candidates for splenectomy, also require chronic RBC transfusion to lower and suppress the concentration of circulating hemoglobin S red cells.[43]

Periodic erythrocytapheresis in sickle cell patients who have had a stroke is effective in minimizing transfusion-related iron overload and prevention of cerebrovascular accidents.[43,44] Chronic transfusion therapy or periodic erythrocytapheresis is also recommended in pediatric and adult sickle cell patients with a history of acute chest syndrome or pulmonary hypertension.[45] Erythrocytapheresis is not recommended for treatment of acute priapism because of its lack of efficacy and concern for neurologic sequelae (ASPEN syndrome: association of sickle cell disease, priapism, exchange transfusion, and neurologic events).[46]

Because chronically transfused patients have a high rate of red cell alloimmunization, it is prudent to perform extended red cell phenotyping or genotyping (including Rh, K, Jk, Fy, Ss) before the first transfusion in such patients.[47] In an effort to prevent red cell antibody formation and repeated delayed hemolytic reactions, many facilities use the extended red cell phenotype to administer partially matched red cells (Rh, K).[43,47] Because of the complexity of the *RH* locus, Rh alloimmunization still occurs despite extended typing.[48] Leukocyte-reduced blood components should be used in chronically transfused patients.[47] These patients generally do not require T-cell inactivated components.

Management of Platelet Refractoriness

Patients who repeatedly fail to achieve a therapeutic increment in platelet count after platelet transfusion are said to be refractory.

The posttransfusion platelet corrected count increment (CCI) can be calculated and used to confirm the development of the refractory state. (See Platelets in Chapter 1: Blood Components.) The onset of refractoriness may be associated with difficulty in controlling clinical bleeding or with repeated febrile reactions to platelet transfusion. In most patients, refractoriness results from nonimmune causes such as infection, fever, splenomegaly, disseminated intravascular coagulation, active bleeding, veno-occlusive disease, and GVHD.[49]

In some patients, refractoriness may be caused by the development of alloantibodies directed against foreign HLA antigens, platelet-specific antigens, ABO incompatibility, or, rarely, drug-induced antibodies. The possibility of ITP or posttransfusion purpura should also be considered. The diagnosis of alloimmunization is supported by a positive test for antibodies to HLA antigens or by a positive platelet crossmatch.

The most common alloantibodies associated with platelet refractoriness are directed against HLA Class I antigens, which are expressed on platelets and all nucleated cells.[49] HLA antibodies develop after exposure to foreign HLA antigens, as may occur during pregnancy, after the transfusion of cellular blood components, and after organ transplantation. Although leukocyte reduction significantly reduces the incidence of primary HLA alloimmunization, it does not prevent a secondary immune response in patients who were previously sensitized through transfusion or pregnancy. (See Chapter 1: Blood Components.)

Effective therapies for alloimmunized patients with severe thrombocytopenia are limited.[49] Platelet transfusions from HLA-unmatched donors are nearly always ineffective, but the use of platelets from HLA-matched donors or family members may restore platelet responsiveness. The extensive polymorphism of the HLA system, however, can preclude the procurement of sufficient HLA-identical donors to meet the needs of refractory patients. The transfusion of platelets from partially or selectively HLA-matched donors may be successful if the match is close enough. Another method for selecting compatible donors compares HLA amino acid sequence information between donor and recipient. Identifying the specificity of the HLA antibody (a process that is analogous to red cell antibody identification) may permit a wider choice of donors with known HLA types.

Platelet crossmatching, in which patient serum/plasma is tested against a panel of single-donor platelets, has also been successful.[49,50] Platelet crossmatching can be extremely helpful when patients do not have an HLA type on record or when there are significant delays in scheduling and obtaining HLA-selected platelets. In addition, direct platelet crossmatching can detect incompatibilities to both HLA and platelet-specific antibodies.[49] Platelet crossmatching is limited by the number of ABO-compatible apheresis platelet units in inventory and the volume of patient serum/plasma available for testing.

In some cases, even the use of well-matched platelets does not result in an adequate posttransfusion increment. Other approaches to managing platelet refractoriness, such as the use of high-dose IVIG, rituximab, therapeutic plasma exchange, splenectomy, splenic irradiation, or epsilon aminocaproic acid, have met with marginal success.[49,51]

Thrombopoietin receptor agonists (romiplostim, eltrombopag), which are approved for treating ITP, have been shown to improve clinical bleeding response in refractory patients by promoting recovery of endogenous platelet production.[52] Eltrombopag is also effective in many patients with thrombocytopenia associated with cirrhosis and chronic liver disease, because it compensates for the low hepatic production of thrombopoietin in these conditions.[53] Thrombocytopenia in the setting of liver cirrhosis can also be managed through partial splenic embolization and laparoscopic splenectomy.[53]

Administration of Blood

The most common cause of fatal hemolytic transfusion reactions is the misidentification of either the blood unit or the recipient.

Among the steps that are necessary for safe transfusion, the positive identification of the patient and of the blood sample is the most critical. After sample collection, identification systems must be in place to ensure that technical and clerical errors are avoided.

At the time of transfusion, the blood component, with the compatibility tag attached (this tag should not be removed), must be compared with the patient's identification bracelet. No discrepancies in spelling or identification numbers should exist. The patient should remain under close observation for 15 minutes after the infusion begins and must be assessed periodically until an appropriate time after the transfusion is completed.[1] In a stable adult, blood components are usually administered over 30 minutes (plasma, platelets) to 120 minutes (RBCs). Blood may be given more slowly in patients who are sensitive to fluid imbalances. As a general rule in stable pediatric patients, blood components are administered at 10 mL/kg over 2 to 3 hours. The infusion rate is dependent on adequate venous access and needle size. For adults, a 20- to 18-gauge needle is appropriate for routine transfusion. In infants and toddlers, the smallest needle for RBC infusion is 24- to 22-gauge, and may require a syringe and pump for administration.

Time Limits for Infusing Blood Components

Blood should be infused within 4 hours and must be started before the expiration time denoted on the unit.[1] If that time is likely to be exceeded, the unit should be divided into aliquots by using a sterile connecting device, and portions should be kept in the blood bank refrigerator until required. A unit of RBCs that has been allowed to warm above 10 C, but is not used, cannot be reissued by the transfusion service. Units that have been washed or otherwise modified may have a shorter expiration time. RBCs and plasma must be stored in monitored refrigerators. Platelets should *never* be refrigerated.

Blood Warming

At routine flow rates, transfused blood does not require warming. The use of blood warmers is generally restricted to the following: rapid and multiple transfusions to adult patients at more than 50 mL/minute for at least 30 minutes; during the patient rewarming phase of cardiopulmonary bypass surgery; exchange transfusions in infants; transfusions to children in volumes ≥ 20 mL/kg/hour; and in cases of severe cold autoimmune hemolytic anemia. Transfusion of cold blood at more than 100 mL/minute has been associated with a higher rate of cardiac arrest than transfusion of warmed blood in a control group.[54]

Most infusion devices have special disposable kits with larger-gauge tubing that are specifically designed for use with the device. In the trauma setting, rapid infusion devices are often integral to blood-warming devices, and they come as a combined instrument. These instruments can rapidly warm and infuse the blood either through peripheral intravenous (IV) catheters of 14- to 18-gauge or central IV catheters of larger diameter. Warming devices mostly use dry heat, but they can also use waterbaths, countercurrent heat exchange, or in-line microwave technology. Modern warmers typically have sensors to tightly compensate for changes in blood flow and to maintain equal warming of blood and other infusibles. Automatic warming devices must have a visible thermometer and should have an audible warning system. Warming the whole unit of blood by immersion in hot water or by using microwave blood warmers is contraindicated because hemolysis can result from overheating.

Infusion Devices

Several electronic infusion devices (ie, blood pumps) are available. These machines are designed to deliver parenteral fluids, including blood components, at flow rates ranging from 0.5 mL/minute to more than 750 mL/minute. The pump mechanisms vary among manufacturers and include syringe-type pumping systems, peristaltic roller devices, and electromechanical pumps that operate on a positive volumetric displacement principle.

Rapid infusion systems can be as simple as an inflatable cuff with a pocket and sphygmomanometer, or they can include electronic instruments that more tightly control the pressure and flow rates. Electronic rapid infusion devices will monitor pressure and compensate to maintain the desired flow without exceeding 300 mm Hg pressure to the bag. Some systems require manufacturer-supplied pump cassettes, whereas others can be used with standard IV administration set tubing. Although most pump systems do not induce mechanical hemolysis when used with Whole Blood, gross hemolysis can result when some models are used to administer RBCs. The manufacturer's insert should be consulted regarding approval for use with blood components. Peak infusion rates and the degree of hemolysis depend on both the infusion device and the sizes of tubing and catheter used.[55,56]

Concomitant Use of Intravenous Solutions

Only normal saline (0.9% USP) and plasmalyte may be administered with blood components. Other solutions may be hypotonic (eg, 5% dextrose in water) and may cause hemolysis in vitro, or they may contain additives such as calcium (lactated Ringer's solution) that can initiate in-vitro coagulation in citrated blood.[57] However, despite some studies showing no increase in coagulation with lactated Ringer's solution, normal saline and plasmalyte remain the only acceptable solutions for mixing with blood components.[57,58] RBCs may be diluted with normal saline to decrease viscosity and increase the infusion rate.

Medications should never be added to a unit of blood or infused with blood, unless the medication is approved for that use by the Food and Drug Administration. Some drugs may cause hemolysis because of their excessively high pH. Furthermore, if medication is added to blood and the transfusion is discontinued for any reason, the dose of infused medication may not be known. Finally, it would be difficult to determine whether any adverse transfusion reactions were caused by the blood or the drug it contained.

Filters

All blood components must be administered through a filter in order to remove blood clots and other debris. Standard blood filters, with a pore size between 170 and 260 microns, trap large aggregates and clots. Microaggregate blood filters with 20- to 40-micron pores can remove microaggregate debris, and they are frequently employed when blood is recirculated in cardiac bypass devices. They are not indicated for routine blood transfusions and do not accomplish leukocyte reduction. Blood filters designed for leukocyte-reduced cellular blood components are available. (See Leukocyte Reduction, Chapter 1: Blood Components.) Disadvantages of both microaggregate and leukocyte reduction filters include the potential to become clogged and the prevention of rapid blood delivery. These problems may be circumvented by using components that have been leukocyte reduced by the blood donor center before issue.

References

1. Ooley PW, ed. Standards for blood banks and transfusion services. 30th ed. Bethesda, MD: AABB, 2016.
2. Butch SH, Oberman HA. The computer or electronic crossmatch. Transfus Med Rev 1997;11:256-64.
3. Padget BJ, Hannon JL. Variations in pretransfusion practices. Immunohematology 2003;19:1-6.
4. Zielinski MD, Schrager JJ, Johnson P, et al. Multicenter comparison of emergency release group A versus AB plasma in blunt-injured trauma patients. Clin Transl Sci 2015;8:43-7.
5. Dutton RP, Shih D, Edelman BB, et al. Safety of uncrossmatched type-O red cells for resuscitation from hemorrhagic shock. J Trauma 2005;59:1445-9.

6. Goodell PP, Uhl L, Mohammed M, Powers AA. Risk of hemolytic transfusion reactions following emergency-release RBC transfusion. Am J Clin Pathol 2010;134:202-6.
7. Gaballa S, Alousi A, Biralt S, Champlin R. Hematopoietic stem cell transplantation. In: Simon TL, McCullough J, Snyder EL, et al, eds. Rossi's principles of transfusion medicine. 5th ed. Chichester, UK: Wiley Blackwell, 2016:440-51.
8. Tay J, Allan DS, Chatelain E, et al. Transfusion of red cells in hematopoietic stem cell transplantation (TRIST): A randomized controlled trial evaluating 2 red cell transfusion thresholds. Blood 2016;22:1032.
9. DeZern AE, Williams K, Zahurak M, et al. Red blood cell transfusion triggers in acute leukemia: A randomized pilot study. Transfusion 2016;56:1750-57.
10. Kaufman RM, Djulbegovic B, Gernsheimer T, et al. Platelet transfusion: A clinical practice guideline from AABB. Ann Intern Med 2015;162:205-13.
11. Stanworth SJ, Estcourt LJ, Poster G, et al. A no-prophylaxis platelet-transfusion strategy for hematologic cancers. N Engl J Med 2013;368:1771-80.
12. Wu A, Buhler LH, Cooper DKC. ABO-incompatible organ and bone marrow transplantation: Current status. Transpl Int 2003;16:291-9.
13. Chung HS, Cho SJ, Park CS. Effects of liver function on ionized hypocalcaemia following rapid blood transfusion. J Int Med Res 2012;40:572-82.
14. Subramanian V, Ramachandran S, Klein C, et al. ABO-incompatible organ transplantation. Int J Immunogenetics 2012;39:282-90.
15. Fehr T, Stussi G. ABO-incompatible kidney transplantation. Curr Opin Organ Transplant 2012;17:376-85.
16. West LJ, Pollock-Barziv SM, Dipchand AI, et al. ABO-incompatible heart transplantation in infants. N Engl J Med 2001;344:793-800.

17. Judd WJ, for the Scientific Section Coordinating Committee. Guidelines for prenatal and perinatal immunohematology. Bethesda, MD: AABB, 2005.
18. Liumbruno GM, D'Alessandro A, Rea F, et al. The role of antenatal immunoprophylaxis in the prevention of maternal-foetal anti-Rh(D) alloimmunization. Blood Transfus 2010;8:8-16.
19. Schonewille H, Klumper FJCM, van de Watering LMG. High additional maternal red cell alloimmunization after Rhesus- and K-matched intrauterine intravascular transfusions for hemolytic disease of the fetus. Am J Obstet Gynecol 2007;196:143e1-e6.
20. Delaney M, Wikman A, van de Watering L, et al. Blood group antigen matching influence on gestational outcomes (AMIGO) study. Transfusion 2017;57:525-32.
21. Moise KJ Jr. Management of rhesus alloimmunization in pregnancy. Obstet Gynecol 2008;112:164-76.
22. De Haas M, Thurik FF, van der Ploeg CPB, et al. Sensitivity of fetal RHD screening for safe guidance of targeted anti-D immunoglobulin prophylaxis: Prospective cohort study of a nationwide programme in the Netherlands. BMJ 2016;355:i5789.
23. Oepkes D, Adama van Scheltema P. Intrauterine fetal transfusions in the management of fetal anemia and fetal thrombocytopenia. Semin Fetal Neonatal Med 2007;12:432-8.
24. Giannina G, Moise KJ Jr, Dorman K. A simple method to estimate volume for fetal intravascular transfusions. Fetal Diagn Ther 1998;13:94-7.
25. Wu Y, Stack G. Blood product replacement in the perinatal period. Semin Perinatal 2007;31;262-71.
26. American Academy of Pediatrics Subcommittee on Hyperbilirubinemia. Clinical practice guidelines: Management of hyperbilirubinemia in the newborn infant 35 or more weeks in gestation. Pediatrics 2004;114:297-316.

27. British Committee for Standards in Haematology. Transfusion guidelines for neonates and older children. Br J Haematol 2004;124:433-53.
28. Arnold DM, Sith JW, Kelton JG. Diagnosis and management of neonatal alloimmune thrombocytopenia. Transfus Med Rev 2008;22:255-67.
29. Peterson JA, McFarland JG, Curtis BR, Aster RH. Neonatal alloimmune thrombocytopenia: Pathogenesis, diagnosis and management. Br J Hematol 2013;161:3-14.
30. Bakchoul T, Bassler D, Heckmann M, et al. Management of infants born with severe neonatal alloimmune thrombocytopenia: The role of platelet transfusions and intravenous immunoglobulin. Transfusion 2014;54:640-5.
31. Strauss RG. Red blood cell transfusion and avoiding hyperkalemia to neonates and infants. Transfusion 2010; 50:1862-5.
32. Crowley M, Kirpalani H. A rational approach to red blood cell transfusion in the neonatal ICU. Curr Opin Pediatr 2010;22:151-7.
33. Christensen RD, Carroll PD, Josephson CD. Evidence-based advances in transfusion practice in neonatal intensive care units. Neonatology 2014;106:245-53.
34. Christensen RD, Baer VL, Lambert DK, et al. Association among very-low-birthweight neonates, between red blood cell transfusions in the week after birth and severe intraventricular hemorrhage. Transfusion 2014;54:104-8.
35. Whyte RK. Neurodevelopmental outcome of extremely low-birth-weight infants randomly assigned to restrictive or liberal hemoglobin thresholds for blood transfusion. Semin Perinatol 2012;36:290-3.
36. Bell EF, Strauss RG, Widness JA, et al. Randomized trial of liberal versus restrictive guidelines for red blood cell transfusion in preterm infants. Pediatrics 2005;115:1685-91.
37. Kirpalani H, Whyte RK, Andersen C, et al. The premature infants in need of transfusion (PINT) study: A randomized, controlled trial of a restrictive (low) versus liberal (high)

transfusion threshold for extremely low birth weight infants. J Pediatr 2006;149:301-7.
38. Liu EA, Mannino FL, Lane TA. Prospective, randomized trial of the safety and efficacy of a limited donor exposure transfusion program for premature neonates. J Pediatr 1994;125:92-6.
39. Lee AC, Reduque LL, Luban NLC, et al. Transfusion-associated hyperkalemic cardiac arrest in pediatric patients receiving massive transfusion. Transfusion 2014;54:244-54.
40. Josephson CD, Caliendo AM, Easley KA, et al. Blood transfusion and breast milk transmission of cytomegalovirus in very low-birth-weight infants: A prospective cohort study. JAMA Pediatr 2014;168:1054-62.
41. Mohan P, Brocklehurst P. Granulocyte transfusions for neonates with confirmed or suspected sepsis and neutropaenia. Cochrane Database Syst Rev 2003;(4):CD003956.
42. Lacroix J, Hébert PC, Hutchison JS, et al. Transfusion strategies for patients in pediatric intensive care units. N Engl J Med 2007;356:1609-19.
43. Roseff SD. Sickle cell disease: A review. Immunohematology 2009;25:67-74.
44. Lee MT, Piomelli S, Granger S, et al. Stroke prevention trial in sickle cell anemia (STOP): Extended follow-up and final results. Blood 2006;108:847-52.
45. Klings ES, Machado RF, Barst RJ, et al. An official American Thoracic Society clinical practice guideline: Diagnosis, risk stratification, and management of pulmonary hypertension of sickle cell disease. Am J Respir Crit Care Med 2014;189:727-40.
46. Kato GJ. Priapism in sickle-cell disease: A hematologist's perspective. J Sex Med 2012;9:70-8.
47. Vichinsky EP, Luban NL, Wright E, et al. Prospective RBC phenotype matching in a stroke-prevention trial in sickle cell anemia: A multicenter transfusion trial. Transfusion 2001;41:1086-92.

48. Chou ST, Jackson T, Vege S, et al. High prevalence of red blood cell alloimmunization in sickle cell disease despite transfusion from Rh-matched minority donors. Blood 2013;122:1062-71.
49. Vassallo R, Fung M. Management of the platelet-transfusion refractory patient. In: Sweeney JD, Lozano M, eds. Platelet transfusion therapy. Bethesda, MD: AABB Press, 2013:321-58.
50. Vassallo RR, Fung M, Rebulla P, et al. Utility of crossmatched platelet transfusions in patients with hypoproliferative thrombocytopenia: A systematic review. Transfusion 2014;54:1180-91.
51. Cid J, Magnano L, Acosta M, et al. Rituximab, plasma exchange and intravenous immunoglobulins as a new treatment strategy for severe HLA alloimmune platelet refractoriness. Platelets 2015;26:190-4.
52. Berthelot-Richer M, Boilard B, Morin A, et al. Romiplostim efficacy in an acute myeloid leukemia patient with transfusion refractory thrombocytopenia. Transfusion 2012;52:739-41.
53. Hayashi H, Beppu T, Shirabe K, et al. Management of thrombocytopenia due to liver cirrhosis: A review. World J Gastroenterol 2014;20:2595-605.
54. Boyan CP, Howland WS. Cardiac arrest and temperature of bank blood. JAMA 1963;183:58-60.
55. Frelich R, Ellis MH. The effect of external pressure, catheter gauge, and storage time on hemolysis in RBC transfusion. Transfusion 2001;41:799-802.
56. Millikan JS, Cain TL, Hansbrough J. Rapid volume replacement for hypovolemic shock: A comparison of techniques and equipment. J Trauma 1984;24:428-31.
57. Ryden SE, Oberman HA. Compatibility of common intravenous solutions with CPD blood. Transfusion 1975;15:250-5.
58. Lorenzo M, Davis JW, Negin S, et al. Can Ringer's lactate be used safely with blood transfusions? Am J Surg 1998;175:308-10.

PATIENT BLOOD MANAGEMENT

Concept of Patient Blood Management

Patient blood management (PBM) is an evidence-based, multidisciplinary approach to optimizing the care of patients who might need transfusion. PBM encompasses all aspects of patient evaluation and clinical management surrounding the transfusion decision-making process, including the optimization of patient red cell mass, the minimization of blood loss, and the application of appropriate transfusion indications. PBM can reduce the need for allogeneic blood transfusions and reduce health-care costs while ensuring that blood components are available for the patients who need them.[1,2]

Establishment of a PBM program requires the use of evidence-based criteria and an implementation process that can create an accountable culture to effect changes. Key factors to consider when establishing a blood management program are data collection regarding transfusion practice, evidence-based criteria for blood transfusion, preoperative anemia management, intraoperative measures to reduce blood transfusion, and multidisciplinary clinical transfusion education.

PBM Program Structure

To be successful, PBM programs should include administration, surgical services, finance, nursing, and information technology personnel. Leadership should include transfusion medicine physicians and clinician champions from specialties utilizing substantial amounts of blood components, with an appointed medical director of the program. Dedicated personnel (transfusion safety officers or PBM coordinators) who oversee daily practice and education have proven useful for consistent safety and education follow-through.[3]

Best practices can be realized with evidence-based guidelines and computerized tools to guide physicians and track usage data. Transfusion policies for red cells, platelets, plasma, and cryoprecipitate may be established at an institutional level and derived from published guidelines or standards.[4-6] Indications for transfusion of blood components, setting thresholds for anemia tolerance, and designing strategies to restrict unnecessary transfusion are all important elements of blood utilization review that can be audited by the transfusion committee. Actionable data can be monitored to provide feedback and improve practices over time. Dashboards, programs that analyze laboratory and clinical data and compare against programmed ideals such as benchmarks, can provide up-to-the-minute information about practice in an easy-to-understand format.[7] Information systems can provide clinical decision support by mapping current laboratory values to blood orders and warning when orders are not supported by laboratory values.[8,9]

Nonsurgical/Preoperative Issues

Evaluating Anemia

The World Health Organization defines anemia as a hemoglobin level less than 13 g/dL in men and less than 12 g/dL in premenopausal, nonpregnant women.[10] Clinical findings suggestive of anemia include palpitations, tachycardia, fatigue, angina, mental status changes, and dyspnea, all of which may suggest tissue hypoxia and cardiovascular decompensation. Preoperative anemia should be identified and treated to minimize the risk of perioperative transfusion. Anywhere from 5% to 75% of preoperative patients are anemic, depending on the surgical group and definition of anemia used.[11] Identification of symptoms of anemia, transfusion history, underlying diseases, dietary deficiencies, and factors that increase the likelihood of bleeding in the perioperative period should be thoroughly investigated.[12,13]

Evaluation of current medications should target those that predispose to perioperative bleeding and anemia, such as nonsteroidal anti-inflammatory agents, antiplatelet agents, and anticoagulants. Personal and family history of unexpected bleeding during or after invasive procedures should also be noted. (See Chapter 3: Hemostatic Disorders.)

The goal of the laboratory workup of anemia is to identify those conditions for which short-term interventions can be implemented for preoperative optimization, such as iron, folate, and vitamin B_{12} deficiencies. Findings suggestive of other conditions require further evaluation with a hematologist. Elective surgery should be delayed until the cause is identified, unless the anemia is related to the condition for which surgery is to be performed.[14]

The initial evaluation includes a complete blood count, peripheral smear, and corrected reticulocyte count to determine whether anemia is a result of loss or destruction of red cells, or a decrease in marrow production.[15] Additional tests include iron, total iron-binding capacity, transferrin saturation, ferritin, serum red cell folate, and serum vitamin B_{12} levels.[13]

Iron Supplementation

The most common cause of asymptomatic anemia in surgical patients is iron deficiency. Patients undergoing orthopedic surgery have received more attention, given the frequency of the procedures and attempts to minimize intraoperative blood transfusions; however, preoperative anemia with iron deficiency is not uncommon in other surgical settings.[16] Oral iron supplementation may be insufficient to achieve rapid correction of iron deficiency anemia.[16-19]

The safety and efficacy of parenteral iron have been demonstrated in multiple studies.[20-24] An intravenous (IV) cumulative iron dose of 1 g will raise the hemoglobin level by approximately 2.0 g/dL; use of IV iron has reported benefits in successfully treating anemia and decreasing transfusion rates.[10,19] The Network for Advancement of Transfusion Alternatives (NATA) recommends that preoperative IV iron be administered to patients with a ferritin level of less than 100 ng/mL, a transferrin saturation less than 20%, or an expected blood loss greater than 1500 mL. The cutoff to avoid further IV iron administration is a ferritin level higher than 300 ng/mL and a transferrin saturation greater than 50%, or when there is acute infection.[25] Iron should be administered within sufficient time (3 to 4 weeks before surgery) to maximize effective erythropoiesis.[24]

The adverse reaction of greatest concern associated with IV iron has been anaphylaxis, which occurs more frequently in combination with high-molecular-weight (HMW) dextran.[26] For this reason, HMW dextran is no longer used in much of the world; low-molecular-weight dextran carries a black-box warning.[27] The remaining IV iron formulations differ primarily on cost, time for infusion, and number of doses for administration.[28]

Adverse drug events (ADEs) with the current IV iron formulations are rare (less than 1% of cases) and include fever, nausea, mild allergic reaction, and pain, as well as serious ADEs such as anaphylactoid and anaphylactic reactions.[29] The risk of adverse effects is minimized by using test doses in naïve patients and decreasing the dose per administration.[28]

Preoperative Use of Erythropoiesis-Stimulating Agents

Routine preoperative use of erythropoiesis-stimulating agents (ESAs) occurs mainly in orthopedic surgery (hip and knee replacements) and in cardiac surgery for patients attempting to avoid blood transfusions.[30] The degree of erythropoiesis shows a dose-response correlation.[31] In studies in iron-replete nonanemic patients, reticulocytosis reportedly occurs after 3 days of treatment with erythropoietin (EPO).[32] It has been shown that EPO increases the reticulocyte life span, especially during the first week after its administration.[33] Concomitant use of iron and folate when using EPO allows appropriate plasma transferrin saturation to promote optimal erythropoiesis.[31]

Dose and Administration

The current recommendation for perioperative use of epoetin alfa as it appears on the package insert is 600 units/kg subcutaneously in 4 doses administered 21, 14, and 7 days before surgery, and on the day of surgery.[34,35] Epoetin alfa is indicated for the treatment of anemic patients (hemoglobin >10 ≤13 g/dL) who are at high risk for perioperative blood loss from elective, noncardiac, nonvascular surgery, to reduce the need for allogeneic blood transfusions.[34,35] Insurance may not provide reimbursement for the treatment of preoperative anemia in cardiac and vascular patients. Thus, a prudent physician will consider optimizing the management of the patient's anemia before the perioperative period for these patient populations.

The weekly ESA dose provides ease of administration and a decreased total dose, which maintains enhanced hematopoietic response. The patient should continue taking concomitant parenteral iron (200 mg iron sucrose or 125 mg ferrous sulfate) along with each dose of epoetin alfa, especially if ferritin levels are less than 100 ng/mL.

Controversies Regarding ESA Therapy

In surgical patients undergoing elective spine surgery, the risk of deep venous thrombosis (DVT) was higher among patients who received ESAs (4.7%) than those who did not (2.1%).[36] An increased risk of venous thromboembolism [relative risk 1.57, 95% confidence interval (CI) 1.31-1.87] and mortality (hazard ratio 1.10, 95% CI 1.01-1.20) was seen in 4610 patients with cancer who received ESAs, vs 3562 controls.[37] A meta-analysis by the NATA showed that the risk of DVT increased with the use of recombinant human EPO (Peto odds ratio 1.66, 95% CI 1.10-2.48).[38]

Use of ESA therapy in patients with active malignancy was found to correlate with significantly less overall survival (OS) rates. In patients with head and neck malignancies, progression-free survival was poorer with epoetin beta than with placebo (adjusted relative risk 1.62, 95% Cl 1.22-2.14; p = 0.0008).[39] In breast cancer patients, OS was 70% in those whose anemia was treated with epoetin alfa compared to 76% OS in those on placebo (p = 0.01).[40]

Targeting normal range hemoglobin (13-15 g/dL) and hematocrit levels (40%-45%) in renal failure patients receiving ESAs has shown poorer outcomes compared to those with a less aggressive target for hemoglobin (10-11.5 g/dL) or hematocrit (30%-33%).[29-31]

In 2007, the FDA issued a black-box warning to have a conservative approach to anemia management in chronic renal failure patients, targeting a hemoglobin level of 10 to 12 g/dL. It recommended the use of EPO in patients with cancer only if they were undergoing active myelosuppressive chemotherapy. The FDA also alerted against the higher risk of mortality, stroke, uncontrolled hypertension, and DVT in patients taking EPO, and recommended prophylactic anticoagulation in perioperative surgical patients treated with epoetin alfa, because of the higher risk of DVT.[41]

Preoperative Autologous Blood Donation

Preoperative autologous blood donation (PAD) is the process of collecting and storing the patient's own blood before surgery. PAD is generally discouraged because it predisposes to preoperative anemia, which increases the risk for transfusion at the time of surgery.[42,43] Recent utilization data reflects this, showing a 55% decline from 2009 to 2011 in autologous collections, with another 50% decline from 2011 to 2013.[44,45] In addition, up to 10% to 20% of patients referred for PAD are unable to successfully donate because of an underlying medical condition (2%-3%)

or adverse reactions and complications associated with donation (6%-17%).[43,46] Autologous units are more expensive than allogeneic units, and the cost may not be reimbursed by insurance. The risk of adverse reactions with autologous blood transfusion is 0.04% to 0.09% and includes volume overload, febrile reactions, allergic reactions, and hemolysis.[43] PAD requires significant pre- and intraoperative coordination, with a higher incidence of administrative errors resulting from out-of-order transfusion (giving allogeneic units before autologous; 20%), clerical errors (0.7%-2%), and unit unavailability because of outdating or shipping issues.[43] PAD may also have an increased risk of bacterial contamination caused by underlying medical conditions of the donor.[43]

The risk of adverse reactions is higher in elderly patients and children younger than 17 years of age.[46,47] For patients weighing less than 110 pounds, it is advisable to limit the volume of blood drawn at each donation to 10% of the patient's total blood volume.[46,47] The hematocrit should be at least 33% (hemoglobin 11.0 g/dL) before each donation.[4] Contraindications to PAD include infection or risk of bacteremia, active seizure disorder, uncontrolled hypertension, aortic stenosis, recent myocardial infarction and stroke, and severe cardiopulmonary disease.[42,43,48] Autologous collection during pregnancy can be performed safely, but it is usually unnecessary.[43] PAD is not recommended for patients undergoing procedures with a low probability (<10%) of requiring transfusion.[42,43] The wastage rate for autologous blood is approximately 60%, which indicates that PAD is frequently unnecessary.[43]

Perioperative Techniques

Surgical Blood Order Schedule

A surgical blood order schedule, often called a maximum surgical blood order schedule (MSBOS) or standard surgical blood order schedule (SSBOS), is a reference that provides guidance as to the number of blood components to order perioperatively for the most common surgical procedures. A review of institutional blood use over time can be used to derive an MSBOS that would account for 90% to 95% of the blood needs for a particular surgery.[49] Most commonly, ordering recommendations are made for Red Blood Cells (RBCs), while some centers will also include plasma ordering recommendations as well.

Benefits of the blood order schedule include application of best practice guidance and standardization of care.[50] Prospective order review can take place so that orders that do not match the blood schedule can be reviewed to ensure the patient needs match the additional blood components requested. An MSBOS can reduce hospital costs by reducing pretransfusion testing, avoiding outdating of blood units, and providing a guide for perioperative blood management.[49,51] Disadvantages include the potential for not considering all patient factors when ordering, and being underprepared on complicated cases. Additionally, if a center has a higher-than-average transfusion rate at baseline, using internal data to build the tool will not correlate with evidence-based practice and will lead to continued above-average transfusion rates. Using data from multiple sources to establish ordering guidelines is recommended to establish best practice. The development and acceptance of blood order schedules for elective surgery require a close working relationship among the transfusion, surgery, and anesthesiology services, and the schedules should be updated periodically. In some institutions, the MSBOS may require the approval of the hospital transfusion committee or its equivalent.

Blood ordering practices can be monitored through the transfusion index [RBC units/patient] and/or crossmatch-to-transfusion (C:T) ratio for a particular procedure or surgeon. Tracking of the transfusion index or C:T ratio helps to identify procedures that may benefit from more targeted blood schedules, while avoiding unnecessary crossmatches for procedures unlikely to require transfusion. In the United States, a C:T ratio of less than 2 or a transfusion index greater than 0.3 to 0.5 for a given procedure is considered appropriate for blood units to be ordered and crossmatched.[49,52]

Acute Normovolemic Hemodilution

Acute normovolemic hemodilution (ANH) refers to the collection of 1 or more whole blood units at the onset of surgery, and reinfusion at the end of the procedure. To prevent hypotension, the volume of blood that is removed is replaced with crystalloid or colloid solutions.[42,43] This technique is most useful in patients with an adequate preoperative hemoglobin level (>10.0 g/dL) who are undergoing procedures associated with large-volume blood loss (1000-1500 mL). Relative contraindications for ANH are severe anemia, active ischemic cardiac disease, a low cardiac ejection fraction (<30%), known coagulopathy, and underlying hemoglobinopathy.[42,43] ANH is considered acceptable by many, but not all, Jehovah's Witness patients.

Following ANH, blood lost during surgery has a lower hematocrit and viscosity, which conserves red cell mass and may improve perfusion to capillary beds. In addition, the reinfused blood provides a source of fresh platelets and clotting factors, which may have been depleted during surgery. Finally, ANH eliminates the costs associated with testing, inventory management, and wastage.[42,43]

The techniques used for ANH must ensure that the blood is collected in a sterile manner and is properly labeled and stored in approved plastic blood-collection bags. ANH units may be held at room temperature for 8 hours from collection. If more time is needed, units may be refrigerated at 1-6 C for a maximum of 24 hours from collection as long as refrigeration began in the first 8 hours.[53]

Close patient monitoring is required to guard against fluid overload.

Intraoperative Blood Recovery

Intraoperative blood recovery, also known as cell salvage, involves the collection and subsequent reinfusion of blood recovered from the operative site or from an extracorporeal circuit.[53] It is often used in conjunction with other blood management interventions.[42,54] Patients can receive their own shed blood, which can decrease the need for allogeneic blood transfusion by 23% to 54%.[54] This technique should be considered when estimated blood loss is 20% or more of the patient's blood volume and the mean transfusion for the procedure exceeds 1 unit. Relative contraindications are infection, malignancy, hemoglobinopathies, cold agglutinins, and the presence of certain contaminants (urine, fat, amniotic fluid, malignant cells) or pharmacologic agents (hypotonic irrigation fluids, clotting agents, catecholamines) in the surgical field.[5,42,43] Blood recovery has been performed safely during obstetric and oncologic surgery, provided that blood is washed and reinfused with a leukocyte reduction filter.[42,55,56] Blood recovered by intraoperative collection cannot be transfused to other patients.

Various types of devices are available for retrieval of blood from the operative site. The recovered blood should be washed and filtered before reinfusion.[42,43] The washing of shed blood is recommended to eliminate complement and other activated factors.[43] Cell-washing devices can prepare the equivalent of 10 units of allogeneic blood per hour for reinfusion to a massively bleeding patient. Blood collected and processed under sterile conditions and washed with 0.9% saline USP can be stored at room temperature for as long as 4 hours from the end of collection, or at 1 to 6 C for as long as 24 hours from the start of collection, provided that refrigeration was begun within 4 hours of the start of collection.[53] A written protocol describing all procedures involved must be maintained.[4]

Point-of-Care Testing

Transfusion decisions vary widely between individuals and institutions, especially during surgery and trauma. Many times, components are transfused without the results of standard laboratory testing because of delayed turnaround times. Core laboratory testing often requires centrifuged serum or plasma specimens that add more time to specimen processing. Point-of-care testing

(POCT) often avoids such delays because the technology permits the use of a greater array of specimen samples such as venous, arterial, and/or capillary sampling of whole blood.[57] Implementation of rapid POCT in surgical applications can help to individualize and direct resuscitation efforts in surgical patients.

The substantial benefits of POCT should be balanced against the drawbacks of many POCT methods—namely, decreased precision and accuracy, narrowed reportable ranges, lack of interface with medical record systems, cost per test, and limited clinical settings that are validated and approved by federal regulation. POCT methods usually fall under waived or moderate complexity categories in the Clinical Laboratory Improvement Amendments (CLIA) regulations. Therefore, care providers should appreciate the importance of both validating POCT methods and understanding their limitations, to avoid misinterpretation of results. In addition, the abundance of POCT manufacturers and methods places immense importance on test method selection.[58] POCT is often overseen by a multidisciplinary committee to effectively manage validation, implementation, and competency.

Viscoelastic Coagulation Monitoring

Viscoelastic testing provides useful data in multiple settings where there is a need to measure the clotting process, beginning with fibrin formation through the lysis of the clot. The assays analyze the viscoelastic properties of whole blood samples under low shear conditions and display results both graphically and numerically. Thromboelastography (TEG) and rotational thromboelastometry (ROTEM) are the most widely available platforms.

In trauma studies, viscoelastic testing has been effective in rapidly detecting most coagulation disorders, which allows for the streamlining of massive transfusion protocols in trauma settings.[59-61] In patients undergoing cardiac surgery, the incorporation and use of viscoelastic testing coupled with transfusion algorithms have been shown to decrease transfusion requirements and postoperative blood loss.[62,63]

Viscoelastic testing has also proven to be effective in managing coagulation when multiple factor deficiencies are involved. Unlike the hereditary hemorrhagic disorders that require single-factor replacement, coagulation management in major perioperative and trauma patients often requires the use of multiple components and factor concentrates. Recent review articles provide an excellent overview of the benefit of viscoelastic-testing-based transfusion algorithms in multiple clinical settings.[64,65] Fibrinolysis, the breakdown of clots by anticoagulation factors, can be detected by these methodologies where there is no rapid comparative test in standard coagulation testing.[65]

TEG and ROTEM devices provide similar information on clot kinetics and strength but use different nomenclature to describe the parameters (Fig 2). The test results from the TEG and ROTEM devices cannot be used interchangeably because different activators at various concentrations are used, resulting in different reference ranges.[66,67]

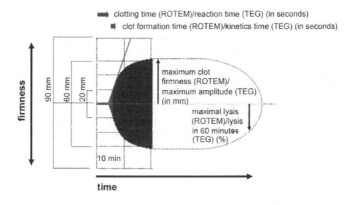

Figure 2. Parameters of viscoelastic or rotational thromboelastometry (eg, ROTEM device, Tem Innovations GmbH, Munich, Germany) and thromboelastography (eg, TEG device, Haemonetics, Braintree, MA).

Abnormal test results should suggest treatment only in the presence of clinically relevant bleeding. However, because the negative predictive value of these POCT analyses is high, a clinically relevant bleeding episode without abnormal test results is most likely of surgical origin. A limitation for both devices is that they are not sensitive enough to detect platelet function disorders or antiplatelet drug effects.

Newer devices perform viscoelastic testing using resonance/sonorheometry methods to produce results that roughly correlate with the above tests.[68,69] In addition, platelet function testing has been evaluated successfully with this methodology and could provide additional utility in assessment of bleeding.[69]

Other Coagulation Monitoring

In addition to viscoelastic testing, the prothrombin time/international normalized ratio (PT/INR), activated clotting time (ACT), and platelet function studies, among others, can be used to monitor coagulation parameters in the surgical suite or intensive care unit.[70] For additional information, see Chapter 3: Hemostatic Disorders.

Many instruments are available for measuring PT/INR, in both waived and moderate complexity test categories, benchtop and handheld models. PT/INR algorithms for PBM often use a PT range of 2.0 × control, or INR 1.5 to 2.0, as decision points for transfusion.[70] Some POCT PT/INR methods have demonstrated decreased accuracy and precision to variable degrees when the INR approaches 1.5 to 4.[71,72] The ACT has been used for many years to monitor heparinization during cardiopulmonary surgery, vascular catheterization, and renal dialysis.[73] The immediate availability of test results can significantly improve clinical care. ACT testing is useful for monitoring large-dose heparin protocols where the activated partial thromboplastin time (aPTT) is too sensitive. ACT testing uses a particulate coagulation activator, usually kaolin or celite. Clotting times are measured in seconds, with a reportable range usually from 50 to 1000 seconds.

Noninvasive testing for continuous hemoglobin monitoring has been used in the intraoperative setting. Although its accuracy has been questioned, the continuous monitor may be useful for trending hemoglobin changes and avoiding wait times for laboratory results.[74,75]

Postoperative Management

Prevention of Excessive Iatrogenic Blood Loss

Decreases in iatrogenic blood losses can be achieved by ordering only essential laboratory tests. These phlebotomy-related blood losses can be minimized by assessment of the patient on a daily basis before determining which laboratory tests are to be ordered (ie, no standing daily laboratory tests). Additional strategies include minimizing the sample volume drawn through the use of pediatric sampling methods and low-volume tubes, maximizing the number of tests to be performed on blood from a single tube, avoiding central venous catheters as access sites, microsampling through POCT, and using noninvasive monitoring whenever possible.[76]

Postoperative Blood Recovery

Collection and reinfusion of shed blood from surgical wounds and drains is one strategy for minimizing the transfusion of allogeneic red cells. This blood is typically defibrinated and unclottable, and it contains high concentrations of fibrinogen-fibrin degradation products, cytokines, activated complement, and cellular proteases.[42,43] In addition, postoperative blood shed from drains is extremely hemodiluted and contains partially hemolyzed red cells. The utility of this technique remains controversial, and its use is limited by both the volume and hematocrit of the shed blood.[43]

Many systems are available; some merely recover shed whole blood for infusion, while others wash and concentrate red cells before infusion. Providers have increasingly favored washed and concentrated red cells for infusion because it has approximately twice the red cell mass per unit volume along with the absence of numerous contaminants, including lipid particles, inflammatory compounds and cytokines, and activated coagulation factors and complement proteins.[42,43] Shed blood must be filtered before reinfusion. Blood intended for reinfusion must be given within 6 hours of the start of collection.[4] Postoperative blood recovery is contraindicated in the presence of local or systemic infection.

Transfusion Thresholds

An anemic patient can tolerate decreased red cell mass variably, depending on multiple parameters, including the rate and volume of blood loss from surgery; heart, kidney, and lung function; hemodynamic stability; and comorbidities. When evaluating a patient with symptomatic anemia, either increasing tolerance for the anemia and/or increasing oxygen-carrying capacity are strategies that can be pursued. Maneuvers to increase tolerance of anemia include medical induction of hypothermia, sedation, paralysis, and maintenance of hemodynamic stability and proper ventilation/oxygenation.

Chapter 4, Transfusion Practices, discusses transfusion thresholds. Outside of the setting of massive hemorrhage or operative procedures with anticipated high-volume blood losses, RBCs should be ordered 1 unit at a time (not 2 or more units at a time).[77] In order to minimize transfusion, patients should be evaluated after each RBC unit is transfused to ascertain whether the specific findings indicative of symptomatic anemia, for which RBC units were initially ordered, have resolved before ordering another unit.

Blood Utilization Review

Ongoing performance improvement efforts known as blood utilization review include a broad range of activities required by accreditation organizations.[78(p92),79-81] Monitoring blood component wastage, patient sample labeling errors, patient identification errors, transfusion deviations, peer review for appropriateness of transfusions, and feedback on practice are several key elements. However, modifying physician ordering practices for transfusion can be challenging. To this end, evidence-based guidelines can be created by the hospital transfusion committee or other peer review groups, and transfusion practices can be monitored periodically. Excursions in practice from established guidelines are opportunities to engage a peer review process and provide feedback to physicians. In addition to adopted guidelines, an individually tailored approach to optimize transfusion management for specific patients in the context of their current medical pictures is important. Differences in patient complexity can have an impact on transfusion requirements. By providing physicians easy access to guidelines and data on their usage, these tools can empower adjustments to habitual patterns of blood ordering and preserve practice autonomy.

The risks of transfusion, its potential impacts on patient outcomes, and its costs are increasingly gaining the attention of accreditation organizations and hospital leadership. This awareness fuels interest in blood utilization review, the development of PBM programs, and the identification of metrics to guide appropriate transfusion practice. Perhaps the most successful strategies for sustained improvement in blood utilization stem from an institutional commitment to change, the identification of departmental stakeholders or divisional champions who might be able to reach individual providers, and both consistency and fairness in the review process by an established peer review group.[82] Because the providers that utilize transfusion for patient management cover a broad range of clinical settings, some tailoring of education to effectively reach the diverse practice environments can be useful. Physician education can take many forms, including seminars, conferences, journal clubs, the results of peer review audits, and one-on-one teaching. In addition, the use of information technology to highlight appropriate indications and provide decision support for best practices, such as requiring documentation of rationale or an alert or warning when laboratory values do not match selected indications, have shown promise in improving blood usage.[83,84]

References

1. Patient blood management. Bethesda, MD: AABB, 2017. [Available at http://www.aabb.org/pbm (accessed July 20, 2017).]
2. Patient blood management learning module: Introduction. Bethesda, MD: AABB, 2014. [Available at http://www.aabb.org/development/learningmodules/Pages/default.aspx (accessed July 20, 2017).]
3. Johnson ST, Puca KE, eds. Transfusion medicine's emerging positions: Transfusion safety officers and patient blood management coordinators. Bethesda, MD: AABB Press, 2013.
4. Holcomb J, ed. Standards for a patient blood management program. 1st ed. Bethesda, MD: AABB, 2014.
5. Berg MP, ed. Standards for perioperative autologous blood collection and administration. 7th ed. Bethesda, MD: AABB, 2016.
6. Carson JL, Grossman BJ, Kleinman S, et al. Red blood cell transfusion: A clinical practice guideline from the AABB. Ann Intern Med 2012;157:49-58.
7. Wintermeyer TL, Liu J, Lee KH, et al. Interactive dashboards to support a patient blood management program

across a multi-institutional healthcare system. Transfusion 2016;56:1480-1.
8. Yazer MH, Triulzi DJ, Reddy V, Waters JH. Effectiveness of a realtime clinical decision support system for computerized physician order entry of plasma orders. Transfusion 2013;53:3120-7.
9. Goodnough LT, Shieh L, Hadhazy E, et al. Improved blood utilization using real-time clinical decision support. Transfusion 2014;54:1358-65.
10. de Benoist B, McLean E, Egli I, Cogswell M, eds. Worldwide prevalence of anaemia 1993-2005: WHO global database on anaemia. Geneva, Switzerland: World Health Organization, 2008. [Available at http://apps.who.int/iris/bitstream/10665/43894/1/9789241596657_eng.pdf (accessed July 20, 2017).]
11. Muñoz M, Gómez-Ramírez S, Kozek-Langeneker S, et al. 'Fit to fly': Overcoming barriers to preoperative haemoglobin optimization in surgical patients. Br J Anaesth 2015;115:15-24.
12. Kumar A, Carson JL. Perioperative anemia in the elderly. Clin Geriatr Med 2008;24:641-8, viii.
13. Kumar A. Perioperative management of anemia: Limits of blood transfusion and alternatives to it. Cleve Clin J Med 2009;76(Suppl 4):S112-18.
14. Goodnough LT, Shander A, Spivak JL, et al. Detection, evaluation, and management of anemia in the elective surgical patient. Anesth Analg 2005;101:1858-61.
15. Mathur SC, Schexneider KI, Hutchison RE. Hematopoiesis. In: McPherson RA, Pincus MR, eds. Henry's clinical diagnosis and management by laboratory methods. 22nd ed. Philadelphia: Saunders-Elsevier, 2011:536-56.
16. Auerbach M, Goodnough LT, Picard D, et al. The role of intravenous iron in anemia management and transfusion avoidance. Transfusion 2008;48:988-1000.
17. MacDougall IC. Iron supplementation in the non-dialysis chronic kidney disease (ND-CKD) patient: Oral or intravenous? Curr Med Res Opin 2010;26:473-82.

18. Goddard AF, James MW, McIntyre AS, et al. Guidelines for the management of iron deficiency anaemia. Gut 2011; 60:1309-16.
19. Lachance K, Savoie M, Bernard M, et al. Oral ferrous sulfate does not increase preoperative hemoglobin in patients scheduled for hip or knee arthroplasty. Ann Pharmacother 2011;45:764-70.
20. Kalantar-Zadeh K, Streja E, Miller JE, et al. Intravenous iron versus erythropoiesis-stimulating agents: Friends or foes in treating chronic kidney disease anemia? Adv Chronic Kidney Dis 2009;16:143-51.
21. Lee TW, Kolber MR, Fedorak RN, et al. Iron replacement therapy in inflammatory bowel disease patients with iron deficiency anemia: A systematic review and meta-analysis. J Crohns Colitis 2012;6:267-75.
22. Muñoz M, Breymann C, García-Erce JA, et al. Efficacy and safety of intravenous iron therapy as an alternative/adjunct to allogeneic blood transfusion. Vox Sang 2008; 94:172-83.
23. Litton E, Xiao J, Ho KM. Safety and efficacy of intravenous iron therapy in reducing requirement for allogeneic blood transfusion: Systematic review and meta-analysis of randomised clinical trials. BMJ 2013;347:f4822.
24. Muñoz M, García-Erce JA, Cuenca J, et al. On the role of iron therapy for reducing allogeneic blood transfusion in orthopaedic surgery. Blood Transfus 2012;10:8-22.
25. Beris P, Muñoz M, García-Erce JA, et al. Perioperative anaemia management: Consensus statement on the role of intravenous iron. Br J Anaesth 2008;100:599-604.
26. McCarthy JT, Regnier CE, Loebertmann CL, et al. Adverse events in chronic hemodialysis patients receiving intravenous iron dextran—a comparison of two products. Am J Nephrol 2000;20:455-62.
27. INFeD package insert. Parsippany, NJ: Actavis Pharma Inc., 2014. [Available at https://www.allergan.com/assets/pdf/infed_pi (accessed July 20, 2017).]

28. Auerbach M, Adamson JW. How we diagnose and treat iron deficiency anemia. Am J Hematol 2016;91:31.
29. Chertow GM, Mason PD, Vaage-Nilsen O, et al. Update on adverse drug events associated with parenteral iron. Nephrol Dial Transplant 2006;21:378-82.
30. Testa U. Erythropoietic stimulating agents. Expert Opin Emerg Drugs 2010;15:119-38.
31. Goodnough LT. Iron deficiency syndromes and iron-restricted erythropoiesis (CME). Transfusion 2012;52: 1584-92.
32. Goodnough LT, Brittenham GM. Limitations of the erythropoietic response to serial phlebotomy: Implications for autologous blood donor programs. J Lab Clin Med 1990; 115:28-35.
33. Krzyzanski W, Perez-Ruixo JJ. An assessment of recombinant human erythropoietin effect on reticulocyte production rate and lifespan distribution in healthy subjects. Pharm Res 2007;24:758-72.
34. Procrit package insert. Horsham, PA: Janssen Products, 2000 (revised May 2012). [Available at http://www.procrit.com/sites/all/themes/procrit/resources/ProcritBooklet.pdf (accessed July 20, 2017).]
35. Epogen package insert. Thousand Oaks, CA: Amgen, 2012. [Available at http://pi.amgen.com/~/media/amgen/repositorysites/pi-amgen-com/epogen/epogen_pi_hcp_english.ashx (accessed July 20, 2017).]
36. Stowell CP, Jones SC, Enny C, et al. An open-label, randomized, parallel-group study of perioperative epoetin alfa versus standard of care for blood conservation in major elective spinal surgery: Safety analysis. Spine (Phila Pa 1976) 2009;34:2479-85.
37. Bennett CL, Silver SM, Djulbegovic B, et al. Venous thromboembolism and mortality associated with recombinant erythropoietin and darbepoetin administration for the treatment of cancer-associated anemia. JAMA 2008;299: 914-24.

38. Goodnough LT, Maniatis A, Earnshaw P, et al. Detection, evaluation, and management of preoperative anaemia in the elective orthopaedic surgical patient: NATA guidelines. Br J Anaesth 2011;106:13-22.
39. Henke M, Laszig R, Rube C, et al. Erythropoietin to treat head and neck cancer patients with anaemia undergoing radiotherapy: Randomised, double-blind, placebo-controlled trial. Lancet 2003;362:1255-60.
40. Leyland-Jones B, Semiglazov V, Pawlicki M, et al. Maintaining normal hemoglobin levels with epoetin alfa in mainly nonanemic patients with metastatic breast cancer receiving first-line chemotherapy: A survival study. J Clin Oncol 2005;23:5960-72.
41. Food and Drug Administration. Information for healthcare professionals: Erythropoiesis stimulating agents (ESA) [Aranesp (darbepoetin), Epogen (epoetin alfa), and Procrit (epoetin alfa)]. (Updated November 8, 2007) Silver Spring, MD: CDER Office of Communications, 2007. [Available at http://www.fda.gov/drugs/drugsafety/postmarketdrug safetyinformationforpatientsandproviders/ucm126481.htm (accessed July 20, 2017).]
42. Waters JH, Frank SM, eds. Patient blood management: Multidisciplinary approaches to optimizing patient care. Bethesda, MD: AABB Press, 2016.
43. McQuilten ZK, Wood EM, Yomtovian RA. Adverse consequences of autologous transfusion practice. In: Popovsky MA, ed. Transfusion reactions. 4th ed. Bethesda, MD: AABB Press, 2012:339-406.
44. US Department of Health and Human Services. The 2011 national blood collection and utilization survey report. Washington DC: DHHS, 2013.
45. Whitaker BI, Rajbhandary S, Harris A. The 2013 AABB blood collection, utilization, and patient blood management survey report. Bethesda, MD: AABB, 2015.
46. Tasaki T, Ohto H. Nineteen years of experience with autotransfusion for elective surgery in children: More troublesome than we expected. Transfusion 2007;47:1503-9.

47. Silvergleid AJ. Safety and effectiveness of predeposit autologous transfusions in preteen and adolescent children. JAMA 1987;257:3403-4.
48. Ferraris VA, Ferraris SP, Saha SP, et al. Perioperative blood transfusion and blood conservation in cardiac surgery: The Society of Thoracic Surgeons and the Society of Cardiovascular Anesthesiologists clinical practice guidelines. Ann Thorac Surg 2007;83:S27-86.
49. Frank SM, Rothschild JA, Masear CG, et al. Optimizing preoperative blood ordering with data acquired from an anesthesia information management system. Anesthesiology 2013;118:1286-97.
50. White MJ, Hazard SW, Frank SM, et al. The evolution of perioperative transfusion testing and blood ordering. Anesth Analg 2015;120:1196-203.
51. Dexter F, Ledolter J, Davis E, et al. Systematic criteria for type and screen based on procedure's probability of erythrocyte transfusion. Anesthesiology 2012;116:768-78.
52. Cheng CK, Trethewey D, Brousseau P, Sadek I. Creation of a maximum surgical blood ordering schedule via novel low-overhead database method. Transfusion 2009;48:2268-9.
53. Waters JH, Dyga RM, Yazer MH, for the Scientific Section Coordinating Committee. Guidelines for blood recovery and reinfusion in surgery and trauma. Bethesda, MD: AABB, 2010.
54. Carless PA, Henry DA, Moxey AJ, et al. Cell salvage for minimizing perioperative allogeneic blood transfusion. Cochrane Database Syst Rev 2010;(4):CD001888.
55. Waters JH, Yazer M, Chen YF, Kloke J. Blood salvage and cancer surgery: A meta analysis of available studies. Transfusion 2012;52:2167-73.
56. Goucher H, Wong CA, Patel SK, Toledo P. Cell salvage in obstetrics. Anesth Analg 2015;121:465-8.
57. Goodnough LT, Hill CC. Use of point-of-care testing for plasma therapy. Transfusion 2012;52(Suppl 1):56S-64S.

58. Dabkowski B. The latest in POC and self testing coag. CAP Today, May 2010.
59. Davenport R, Khan S. Management of major trauma haemorrhage: Treatment priorities and controversies. Br J Haematol 2011;155:537-48.
60. Theusinger OM, Spahn DR, Ganter MT. Transfusion in trauma: Why and how should we change our current practice? Curr Opin Anaesthesiol 2009;22:305-12.
61. Meyer AS, Meyer MA, Sorensen AM. Thromboelastography and rotational thromboelastometry early amplitudes in 182 trauma patients with clinical suspicion of severe injury. J Trauma Acute Care Surg 2014;76:682-90.
62. Ak K, Isbir CS, Tetik S, et al. Thromboelastography-based transfusion algorithm reduces blood product use after elective CABG: A prospective randomized study. J Card Surg 2009;24:404-10.
63. Karkouti K, Callum J, Wijeysundera DN, et al. Point-of-care hemostatic testing in cardiac surgery: A stepped-wedge clustered randomized controlled trial. Circulation 2016;134:1152-62.
64. Wikkelsø A, Wetterslev J, Møller AM, Afshari A. Thromboelastography (TEG) or thromboelastometry (ROTEM) to monitor haemostatic treatment versus usual care in adults or children with bleeding. Cochrane Database Syst Rev 2016;(8):CD007871.
65. Whiting D, DiNardo JA. TEG and ROTEM: Technology and clinical applications. Am J Hematol 2014;89:228-32.
66. Solomon C, Sorensen B, Hochleitner G. Comparison of whole blood fibrin-based clot tests in thromboelastography and thromboelastometry. Anesth Analg 2012;114:721-30.
67. Venema LF, Post WJ, Hendriks HG, et al. An assessment of clinical interchangeability of TEG and ROTEM thromboelastographic variables in cardiac surgical patients. Anesth Analg 2010;111:339-44.
68. Reynolds, PS, Middleton P, McCarthy H, Spiess BD. A comparison of a new ultrasound-based whole blood visco-

elastic test (SEER Sonorheometry) versus thromboelastography in cardiac surgery. Anesth Analg 2016;123:1400-7.
69. Dias JD, Haney EI, Mathew BA, et al. New-generation thromboelastography: Comprehensive evaluation of citrated and heparinized blood sample storage effect on clot-forming variables. Arch Pathol Lab Med 2017;141: 569-77.
70. Abeysundara L, Mallett SV, Clevenger B. Point-of-care testing in liver disease and liver surgery. Semin Thromb Hemost 2017;43:407-15.
71. Karon BS, McBane RD, Chaudhry R, et al. Accuracy of capillary whole blood international normalized ratio on the CoaguCheck S, CoaguCheck XS, and i-STAT 1 point- of-care analyzers. Am J Clin Pathol 2008;130:88-92.
72. Green TL, Mansoor A, Newcommon N, et al. Reliability of point-of-care testing of INR in acute stroke. Can J Neurol 2008;35:348-51.
73. Doty DB, Knott HW, Hoyt JL, et al. Heparin dose for accurate anticoagulation in cardiac surgery. J Cardiovasc Surg 1979;20:597-604.
74. Berkow L, Rotolo S, Mirski E. Continuous noninvasive hemoglobin monitoring during complex spine surgery. Anesth Analg 2011;113:1396-402.
75. Rice MJ, Gravenstein N, Morey TE. Noninvasive hemoglobin monitoring: How accurate is enough? Anesth Analg 2013;117:902-7.
76. Sanchez-Giron F, Alvarez-Mora F. Reduction of blood loss from laboratory testing in hospitalized adult patients using small-volume (pediatric) tubes. Arch Pathol Lab Med 2008;132:1916-19.
77. AABB. Choosing wisely: Five things physicians and patients should question. Philadelphia, PA: ABIM Foundation, 2014. [Available at https://www.aabb.org/pbm/Documents/Choosing-Wisely-Five-Things-Physicians-and-Patients-Should-Question.PDF (accessed July 20, 2017)].
78. Ooley PW, ed. Standards for blood banks and transfusion services. 30th ed. Bethesda, MD: AABB, 2016.

79. Rhamy JF. Synergies between blood center and hospital quality systems. Transfusion 2010;50:2793-7.
80. Patient blood management performance measures project. Oakbrook Terrace, IL: The Joint Commission, 2011. [Available at http://www.jointcommission.org/patient_blood_management_performance_measures_project/ (accessed July 20, 2017).]
81. College of American Pathologists, Commission on Laboratory Accreditation. Transfusion medicine checklist. July 28, 2015 ed. Northfield, IL: CAP, 2015.
82. Puca KE. Patient blood management. In: Fung MK, Eder AF, Spitalnik SL, Westhoff CM, eds. Technical manual. 19th ed. Bethesda, MD: AABB, 2017;20:527-56.
83. Lam H-TC, Schweitzer SO, Petz MH, et al. Effectiveness of a prospective physician self-audit transfusion-monitoring system. Transfusion 1997;37:577-84.
84. Fernandez Perez ER, Winters JL, Gajic O. The addition of decision support into computerized physician order entry reduces red blood cell transfusion resource utilization in the intensive care unit. Am J Hematol 2007;82:631-3.

BLOOD COMPONENT RESUSCITATION IN TRAUMA AND MASSIVE BLEEDING

Introduction

The approach to the massively bleeding patient must be prompt, coordinated, multifaceted, interdisciplinary, and evidence-based. The optimal management of patients requiring massive transfusion (MT) must include not only volume resuscitation and blood component transfusion, but also the judicious and appropriate use of laboratory tests and adjunctive therapies, such as antifibrinolytics. (See Prohemostatic Drugs in Chapter 3: Hemostatic Disorders.) Data-driven transfusion policies and protocols, continuing education of clinical and laboratory staff, and effective communication between clinical teams, the transfusion medicine service, and the laboratory are critical to the successful implementation and deployment of services in the setting of MT.

Traditionally, MT has been defined as the transfusion of 10 or more Red Blood Cell (RBC) units, or approximately the total blood volume (TBV) of an average adult patient, within a 24-hour period.[1,2] Although this definition proved useful for retrospective studies investigating patient outcomes, it has been of little use in the triage of exsanguinating patients. Two more pragmatic definitions are: 1) transfusion of 4 RBC units in 1 hour with anticipation of a continued need for component support,[3] and 2) replacement of 50% of the TBV within 4 hours.[4] In the pediatric population, MT definitions are usually based on the percentage of the TBV transfused, and ongoing hemorrhage of greater than 10% TBV/minute is one widely used indicator.[5]

Among injured civilian patients admitted to trauma centers, it has been estimated that up to 40% of trauma-related mortality is the result of uncontrolled or refractory hemorrhage, and 3% to 5% of these trauma patients require MT.[6,7] Although usually discussed in the setting of the bleeding trauma patient, the need for MT can also occur in medical and surgical settings and in cases of obstetric hemorrhage, where it represents the most common cause of maternal mortality worldwide.[8,9]

Hemostatic Resuscitation in Massive Bleeding

The goals of hemostatic resuscitation in the massively bleeding patient are manifold: control of bleeding, replacement of circulating volume, restoration of tissue oxygenation, correction of coagulopathy, and management of the acute and delayed complications, including electrolyte imbalances, acidosis, hypothermia, and potentially infection. Of particular concern in the bleeding trauma patient is the relatively high (16%-24%) incidence of early trauma-induced coagulopathy (ETIC), which results from the dysregulation of multiple procoagulant, anticoagulant, and fibrinolytic pathways and is independent of the dilutional effects of fluid and component resuscitation.[10,11]

The key components of managing the hemorrhaging trauma patient include damage control surgery and damage control resuscitation, a concept that involves minimizing hypothermia and acidosis and reversing the effects of ETIC. In the initial stages of resuscitation, overzealous resuscitation with crystalloid and colloid fluids leads to increased arterial pressure, potentially causing clot disruption and exacerbation of bleeding, as well as leading to dilution of red cells, platelets, and coagulation factors, and contributing to hypothermia. In addition, these fluids may have proinflammatory effects on the endothelial glycocalyx resulting in increased fluid extravasation.[12,13] As a result, there has been a paradigm shift towards permissive hypotension, early use of blood components, and limiting the volume of crystalloid administered.[14]

Massive Transfusion Protocol

A massive transfusion protocol (MTP) is a system for rapidly providing blood components for exsanguinating patients. MTPs aim to standardize the approach to massively bleeding patients by formalizing an institutional response procedure, systematizing communication pathways, ensuring facilities are in place for frequent laboratory monitoring, and reducing delays in ordering and transportation of blood components to the patient's bedside. As such, MTPs are usually developed, implemented, and monitored by a multidisciplinary team including physicians, nurses, and laboratory staff.

A recent study involving three level-1 trauma centers in the United States has shown that the majority of MTP activations occurred in the emergency department or operating room (84%-95%), and the main indication for MTP activation was trauma-induced bleeding.[15] Retrospective data from trauma patients suggest improved survival after implementation of institutional MTPs, but these studies are limited by their design.[16-18] The improved patient survival may be attributed to improved communication between the clinical staff and the transfusion service and/or optimization of blood component availability and delivery.[19-21] MTPs have become commonplace in both the trauma and nontrauma settings in the United States and in other developed countries. They provide rapid access to blood components in a systematized and standardized manner that simplifies the ordering of components in an emergency while minimizing wastage.[20] Few studies have evaluated the benefits of MTP implementation in the nontrauma setting, but in general, there are no unique disadvantages of using them in this population from the resource allocation perspective, with the potential advantage that components are issued more quickly and with less variability.[22,23]

Blood Component Transfusion Strategies in Massive Hemorrhage

Fixed-Ratio Component Transfusion

A fixed-ratio component transfusion (FRCT) strategy attempts to recapitulate the contents of whole blood using blood components. One of the first papers to suggest a survival benefit from FRCT evaluated the overall mortality of 246 patients receiving MT at an army combat support hospital. There was significantly longer survival among those who received a higher ratio (ie, closer to 1:1) of plasma to RBCs. However, survivor bias likely had a major impact on this result; that is, patients who lived longer because they were less severely injured received more plasma.[24]

The Prospective, Observational, Multicenter, Major Trauma Transfusion (PROMMTT) study was an initial attempt to prospectively examine the relationship of in-hospital mortality to early transfusion of plasma and/or platelets and to plasma:RBC and platelet:RBC ratios during the first 6 hours of resuscitation at 10 level-1 trauma centers in the United States.[25] The investigators found that employing a low plasma:RBC transfusion ratio (<1:2) was associated with increased mortality only in the first 24 hours after admission, but the subsequent risk of death at 30 days was not related to the plasma- or platelet-to-RBC ratio. The Pragmatic Randomized Optimal Platelet and Plasma Ratios (PROPPR) study is the largest randomized trial on FRCT.[26] This study found no differences in the primary outcomes of 24-hour and 30-day all-cause mortality in the 680 patients who were randomly assigned to receive plasma, platelets, and RBCs in a 1:1:1 ratio vs a 1:1:2 ratio. Several secondary outcome differences were present between these two groups and favored the 1:1:1 ratio group, including exsanguination as the primary cause of death within 24 hours of admission and achieving anatomical hemostasis. This study also had some limitations, including the absence of a control arm where the patients would have been resuscitated using something other than an FRCT strategy. Thus, while the two FRCT arms produced similar results, evidence for the ultimate technique for resuscitating MT patients remains elusive.

In nontrauma patients who are receiving MT, there appears to be no significant difference in survival between patients receiving higher ratios of plasma:RBCs or platelets:RBCs and those receiving lower ratios.[27,28] Further research into FRCT in the massively bleeding nontrauma patient is required before making conclusions about the optimal transfusion strategy in these patients.

Goal-Directed Component Therapy

Goal-directed component therapy (GDCT) is a lean approach to MT with the aim of replacing exactly what the patient is lacking, while attempting to minimize over- and undertransfusion, wastage, and potential complications from transfusion. Laboratory tests in GDCT are essential, because they form the basis for transfusion decision making. Turnaround times may limit the utility of the complete blood count (CBC), prothrombin time (PT), activated partial thromboplastin time (aPTT), and fibrinogen assays in real time. Viscoelastic tests (VETs) such as thromboelastography (TEG) and rotational thromboelastometry (ROTEM), when offered at the point of care, significantly shorten turnaround time to 10 to 30 minutes and provide actionable data on coagulation factor status, platelet count and function, and the presence of hyperfibrinolysis.[29] Transfusion algorithms for TEG and ROTEM have been published.[30-32]

Based on the available evidence, a reasonable approach to a massively bleeding patient is to initiate an FRCT strategy in the early stages of damage control resuscitation, because it emphasizes plasma replacement for the significant minority of trauma patients who are coagulopathic upon presentation in the emergency department, and to transition to a GDCT strategy as results of VETs and conventional coagulation assays become available.

Operational Aspects of an MTP

As outlined in the American College of Surgeons' Trauma Quality Improvement Program (ACS-TQIP),[33] the major components of an MTP include: a written protocol outlining the triggers for activating an MTP and who is authorized to activate it; a mechanism for notification of the transfusion service/blood bank and laboratory regarding the activation and deactivation of an MTP; a laboratory testing algorithm for analysis of the patient's blood group and antibody screen, CBC, PT, aPTT, fibrinogen activity, and blood gases, including details regarding specimen collection and transportation and transfusion targets; blood component preparation and delivery guidelines including predetermined MTP package contents; the use of adjunctive therapies; and performance improvement monitoring. (See Fig 3.)

When Should an MTP Be Activated?

Early recognition and treatment of the massively bleeding patient is associated with improved survival outcomes. However, it can be difficult to predict which hemorrhaging patient may eventually require MT. In a survey of trauma centers participating in the ACS-TQIP, all sites reported that they used trauma surgeon judgment as a trigger for MTP activation, with hypotension and administration of uncrossmatched blood components used as a trigger about half of the time.[34] The Trauma-Associated Severe Hemorrhage (TASH) score is a composite score used to predict the need for 10 or more RBC units within a 24-hour period.[35] Other scoring systems that have been developed and validated in the trauma setting include the Assessment of Blood Consumption (ABC) score and the Prince of Wales Hospital (PWH) score.[36,37] Attempts to develop scoring systems have also been made in the liver transplantation and cardiac surgery set-

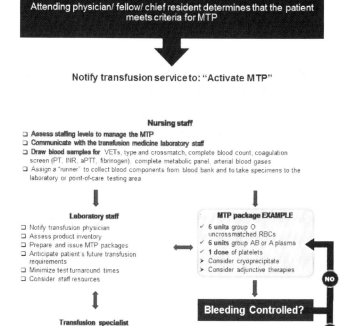

Figure 3. Sample massive transfusion protocol (MTP) algorithm. Note that the contents of the MTP package vary by institution. VETs = viscoelastic tests; PT = prothrombin time; INR = international normalized ratio; aPTT = activated partial thromboplastin time; RBCs = Red Blood Cells.

tings.[38,39] The obstetric shock index (pulse rate divided by systolic blood pressure) has shown utility in identifying significant blood loss in patients with massive postpartum hemorrhage (PPH); a score greater than 1 is associated with massive hemorrhage.[40] Table 12 shows select prediction tools for MT in the civilian posttrauma setting.

MTP Packages

The MTP provides the clinical team with rapid access to a significant quantity of RBCs, plasma, and platelets during the resuscitation, to be transfused as necessary. In trauma centers, group O uncrossmatched RBCs are generally stored in an easily accessible location in the trauma bay, with or without thawed plasma. In other settings, the blood bank issues group O uncrossmatched RBCs and plasma (in coolers) and platelets to transportation personnel, or a pneumatic tube system is used. Blood components are automatically issued in rounds containing predetermined quantities of components until the MTP is deactivated or the patient no longer requires transfusion. The contents of these packages and accompanying adjunct therapies vary from institution to institution.

In the early stages of resuscitation upon meeting MTP triggers, the ACS-TQIP guidelines recommend transfusion of RBC and plasma components in a ratio between 1:1 and 1:2, along with one apheresis platelet unit or a dose of whole-blood-derived platelets for every 6 units of RBCs.[33] The guidelines state that rounds of MTP packages should be delivered at 15-minute intervals until the MTP is terminated, with a goal of the transfusion service having at least one MTP round available for the duration of the MTP activation. The ACS-TQIP also stipulates that designated trauma centers and their supporting blood banks should maintain in inventory the following blood components for immediate release as part of an MTP: at least 8 units of uncrossmatched group O RBCs and at least 8 units of thawed AB or low-titer group A plasma, with additional plasma available within 15 minutes of MTP activation.[33]

Safety of Using Group O Uncrossmatched RBCs

When the recipient's ABO group is unknown, uncrossmatched group O RBCs are issued, because they will be compatible with

Table 12. Prediction Tools for Massive Transfusion in the Civilian Post-trauma Setting[35,36,38]

	TASH score		ABC score	
	Criteria	Score	Criteria	Score
Demographic	Male gender	1		
Clinical	HR > 120 b/min	2	SBP < 90 mm Hg	1
	Free abdominal fluid	3	HR > 120 b/min	1
	Clinically unstable pelvic fracture	6	Penetrating mechanism	1
	Open or dislocated femur fracture	3	Positive FAST	1
Laboratory	Hb < 7 g/dl	8		
	Hb < 9 g/dl	6		
	Hb < 10 g/dl	4		
	Hb < 11 g/dl	3		
	Hb < 12 g/dl	2		
	Base excess < –10	4		
	Base excess < –6	3		
	Base excess < –2	1		
Threshold		≥18		≥2

TASH = Trauma-Associated Severe Hemorrhage; ABC = Assessment of Blood Consumption; HR = heart rate (beats per minute); SBP = systolic blood pressure; FAST = focused abdominal sonography for trauma; Hb = hemoglobin.

the recipient's preformed A and/or B antibodies. The risk of a hemolytic transfusion reaction from receiving uncrossmatched RBCs is very low, even in patients with unexpected antibodies directed against minor red cell antigens (ie, not A or B antigens).[41] In one study of 581 uncrossmatched group O RBCs transfused to 161 patients, no acute hemolytic transfusion reactions were identified.[42] Another study noted a very low (0.4%) incidence of acute hemolysis following transfusion of group O uncrossmatched RBCs to 262 patients.[43,44] Thus, in a hemodynamically unstable trauma patient, it is safe to use uncrossmatched group O RBCs in the resuscitation. Lifesaving uncrossmatched RBCs should not be withheld from a massively bleeding patient while awaiting the results of ABO typing and compatibility testing.

Transition to Group-Specific Blood Components

Samples for ABO blood group determination, antibody screen, and RBC crossmatch should be sent to the blood bank as soon as possible and preferably before the patient receives uncrossmatched RBCs. This will prevent overutilization of group O RBCs and group AB plasma inventories if the patient's ABO group cannot be determined because of the patient's receipt of large quantities of O RBCs. Some centers have a policy requiring a check-group sample on a patient without a historical ABO group on file as a safeguard to detect wrong blood in tube (WBIT) miscollections, which are a major cause of ABO mismatched transfusions in the high-stress setting of a massively bleeding patient.[45] Uncrossmatched ABO-group-specific components are usually available from the blood bank within 10 to 15 minutes of receiving the ABO typing sample(s). Crossmatched RBCs can usually be issued within an hour of the transfusion service receiving the recipient's samples if an unexpected antibody is not detected on the antibody screening panel. If an unexpected antibody is detected (in approximately 5% of transfusion recipients[46]), further laboratory evaluation, including identification of the antibody and finding compatible RBC units, may take several hours to days to complete. In the United States, platelets are generally transfused without regard to donor and recipient ABO groups, so ABO-group-specific platelets are not issued in most adult settings.

Special Considerations: Use of RhD-Positive Components in RhD-Negative or RhD-Status-Unknown Patients

In general, D-negative group O uncrossmatched RBCs are used preferentially in the initial resuscitation of females of childbearing potential because of the risk of D-alloimmunization (up to 21% for RBCs and 1.4% for platelets) and its potential for causing hemolytic disease of the fetus and newborn (HDFN).[47-49] Each institution is required by AABB standards to have a clearly defined policy for the use of D-positive components in D-negative patients,[50(p37)] and this should be extended to those in whom the D status is unknown at the time of transfusion. In order to preserve the blood component inventory, transfusion services may switch massively bleeding D-negative or status-unknown men and women to D-positive components on a case-by-case basis.

Special Considerations: Thawed Plasma, Liquid Plasma, and Low-Titer Group A Plasma

In the MT setting, plasma is the preferred fluid for combined volume resuscitation and replenishment of coagulation factors.[51] Administration of either Fresh Frozen Plasma (FFP), which is frozen within 8 hours of collection, or Plasma Frozen Within 24 Hours After Phlebotomy (PF24) is acceptable, and both components can be thawed and stored for up to 24 hours.[52] The availability of Thawed Plasma, which can be stored for up to 5 days in a refrigerator, in hospital emergency departments and blood banks also permits the immediate and early administration of plasma to massively bleeding patients. Liquid (or never-frozen) Plasma is stored at 1 to 6 C for up to 26 days and maintains coagulation factor levels that are comparable to Thawed Plasma for the first 7 days of storage, with a subsequent decline in levels thereafter.[53,54] It has been approved by the Food and Drug Administration for the initial treatment of patients who are undergoing MT because of life-threatening trauma/hemorrhages and who have clinically significant coagulation deficiencies.[55]

With the widespread adoption of MTPs, there has been a renewed focus on the use of low-titer group A plasma, because of the limited supply of AB plasma. The safety of this practice can be inferred from the very low rate of hemolysis following the transfusion of apheresis platelets, which contain approximately the same amount of plasma as a plasma unit,[52,56] and from the results of the Safety of the Use of Group A Plasma in Trauma (STAT) study, which showed no increase in in-hospital or early (<24 hours after admission) mortality, or hospital length of stay, between group A vs B and AB trauma patients who were resuscitated with at least 1 unit of group A plasma.[57]

Special Considerations: Use of Cold-Stored Whole Blood

There has been a resurgence of interest in the use of cold-stored whole blood (cWB) for the management of civilian trauma patients, although its availability is currently limited. The advantages of cWB over component therapy include less dilution of cellular and plasma components because of a lower volume of additive and anticoagulant solutions; fewer donor exposures; and the opportunity to simplify the logistics of damage control resuscitation. In-vitro studies have shown that platelet function in cWB is comparable to platelets stored at room temperature, without the need for agitation.[58-62] Additionally, cWB units with low titers of both anti-A and -B may be selected for transfusion to mitigate the risk of immediate ABO-mediated hemolysis caused by a minor mismatch.[47,63] cWB has the potential to be the ideal prehospital resuscitation blood component because it is stored and transported in the same way as conventional RBC units, provides some plasma that is essential early in the resuscitation, and has additional hemostatic benefit, since it also contains some functional platelets.

Special Considerations: Obstetric Hemorrhage

Obstetric hemorrhage occurs mainly after delivery, when it is referred to as PPH. The annual incidence of PPH worldwide is estimated at between 4% and 6%, and PPH is a leading cause of pregnancy-associated death.[9] There is no universal definition of PPH, with criteria ranging from an estimated blood loss of >500 mL with vaginal delivery to >1000 mL with cesarean delivery, a decrease in hematocrit by more than 10%, hemodynamic instability, or merely the need for blood transfusion. PPH can occur at delivery or may be delayed, sometimes occurring days after delivery. PPH risk factors include uterine atony, retained placenta, placenta previa and accreta, fetal death, trauma, and acquired or congenital coagulation disorders.[9]

In general, the transfusion management of PPH follows the same guidelines as for other instances of massive bleeding. PPH may require more aggressive cryoprecipitate support, based on studies suggesting a link between PPH and fibrinogen <200 mg/dL.[64] In addition, these patients may receive pharmacologic agents to improve uterine tone.[65] An international, randomized, double-blind, placebo-controlled trial has shown that tranexamic acid reduced death from bleeding in women with PPH, especially if given early, with no significant increase in adverse effects.[66] PPH that is refractory to medical and transfusion management may require uterine tamponade, uterine compression, pelvic vessel embolization, or hysterectomy.[65]

MTP Performance Improvement Monitoring

The ACS-TQIP guidelines recommend monitoring of the following MTP key performance indicators: time from MTP activation to infusion of the first RBC unit and the first plasma unit; adherence to a predetermined FRCT strategy between 1 and 2 hours after MTP activation; deactivation of the MTP by informing the transfusion service within 1 hour of termination of the protocol; and wastage rates for blood components.[33] Although only about 60% to 70% of RBCs and plasma units and 25% of platelets issued in MTP packages are actually transfused, wastage rates remain relatively low (0-9% for RBCs, 0-7% for plasma and platelets, and 7-33% for cryoprecipitate), as evidenced by one retrospective study of three level-1 trauma centers.[15] There is a delicate balance between apportioning a significant quantity of components for a single patient who might not receive them all and ensuring clinicians have all the components that they need when resuscitating exsanguinating patients. However, given the low wastage rates, overissuing components in massive bleeding situations would seem more prudent than underissuing. Nonetheless, it is important that the hospital transfusion service actively monitor component return and wastage rates associated with MTP activations in order to further tailor the protocol to the practice habits and needs of clinicians.

Adjunctive Therapies in MT

Pharmacologic agents provide additional hemostatic capacity and can be employed in MTPs to address underlying coagulopathic processes. Although the strongest evidence for the utility of incorporating a pharmacologic agent into MTPs exists for tranexamic acid, other medications have also been investigated.

Tranexamic acid inhibits fibrinolysis by reversibly antagonizing the lysine-binding site on plasminogen and plasmin.[67] Tranexamic acid can mitigate the effects of primary hyperfibrinolysis, which has been reported in 34% of trauma patients requiring MT.[68,69] The Clinical Randomisation of an Antifibrinolytic in Significant Haemorrhage 2 (CRASH-2) trial demonstrated the efficacy of early administration of tranexamic acid in reducing mortality.[70] The greatest benefit in reducing the risk of death from bleeding occurred if it was administered within 1 hour of injury, and a smaller mortality reduction occurred if it was administered within 1 to 3 hours. There was no increase in vaso-occlusive events, but treatment with tranexamic acid after 3 hours from the time of injury was associated with worse outcomes and appeared to increase the risk of death from bleeding. The CRASH-2 trial used a 1-gram loading dose administered intravenously over 10 minutes followed by an infusion of 1 gram over 8 hours. The use of a fixed dose in trauma situations is more practical than determining dosage by weight for a critically injured patient.

There is limited evidence at present to recommend the routine use, in MT protocols, of fibrinogen concentrates, desmopressin (a synthetic analogue of the antidiuretic hormone vasopressin), and prothrombin complex concentrates (PCCs), which consist of various combinations and concentrations of Factors II, VII, IX, and X, and proteins C and S.[71-73] As for activated recombinant Factor VII (rFVIIa), prospective studies have shown that the use of rFVIIa may decrease the overall need for blood components in trauma patients.[74,75] However, there is no evidence of a survival benefit in the treatment of trauma-related hemorrhage, there are concerns about an increased incidence of arterial thromboembolic events, and the high cost of the product limits its availability.[76-78] As a result, rFVIIa is no longer recommended as an adjunctive therapy in MTPs.[79]

References

1. Raymer JM, Flynn LM, Martin RF. Massive transfusion of blood in the surgical patient. Surg Clin North Am 2012;92: 221-34, vii.
2. Sharpe JP, Weinberg JA, Magnotti LJ, et al. Toward a better definition of massive transfusion: Focus on the interval of hemorrhage control. J Trauma Acute Care Surg 2012; 73:1553-7.
3. Moren AM, Hamptom D, Diggs B, et al. Recursive partitioning identifies greater than 4 units of packed red blood cells per hour as an improved massive transfusion definition. J Trauma Acute Care Surg 2015;79:920-4.
4. Mitra B, Cameron PA, Gruen RL, et al. The definition of massive transfusion in trauma: A critical variable in exam-

ining evidence for resuscitation. Eur J Emerg Med 2011; 18:137-42.
5. Diab YA, Wong EC, Luban NL. Massive transfusion in children and neonates. Br J Haematol 2013;161:15-26.
6. Sauaia A, Moore FA, Moore EE, et al. Epidemiology of trauma deaths: A reassessment. J Trauma 1995;38:185-93.
7. Como JJ, Dutton RP, Scalea TM, et al. Blood transfusion rates in the care of acute trauma. Transfusion 2004;44:809-13.
8. McLintock C, James AH. Obstetric hemorrhage. J Thromb Haemost 2011;9:1441-51.
9. Oyelese Y, Ananth CV. Postpartum hemorrhage: Epidemiology, risk factors, and causes. Clin Obstet Gynecol 2010; 53:147-56.
10. MacLeod JB, Winkler AM, McCoy CC, et al. Early trauma induced coagulopathy (ETIC): Prevalence across the injury spectrum. Injury 2014;45:910-15.
11. Brohi K, Singh J, Heron M, Coats T. Acute traumatic coagulopathy. J Trauma 2003;54:1127-30.
12. Neal MD, Hoffman MK, Cuschieri J, et al. Crystalloid to packed red blood cell transfusion ratio in the massively transfused patient: When a little goes a long way. J Trauma Acute Care Surg 2012;72:892-8.
13. Duchesne JC, Heaney J, Guidry C, et al. Diluting the benefits of hemostatic resuscitation: A multi-institutional analysis. J Trauma Acute Care Surg 2013;75:76-82.
14. Kutcher ME, Kornblith LZ, Narayan R, et al. A paradigm shift in trauma resuscitation: Evaluation of evolving massive transfusion practices. JAMA Surg 2013;148:834-40.
15. Dunbar NM, Olson NJ, Szczepiorkowski ZM, et al. Blood component transfusion and wastage rates in the setting of massive transfusion in three regional trauma centers. Transfusion 2017;57:45-52.
16. Riskin DJ, Tsai TC, Riskin L, et al. Massive transfusion protocols: The role of aggressive resuscitation versus product ratio in mortality reduction. J Am Coll Surg 2009;209: 198-205.

17. Cotton BA, Au BK, Nunez TC, et al. Predefined massive transfusion protocols are associated with a reduction in organ failure and postinjury complications. J Trauma 2009;66:41-8; discussion 8-9.
18. Zaydfudim V, Dutton WD, Feurer ID, et al. Exsanguination protocol improves survival after major hepatic trauma. Injury 2010;41:30-4.
19. Meyer DE, Vincent LA, Fox EE, et al. Every minute counts: Time to delivery of initial massive transfusion cooler and its impact on mortality. J Trauma Acute Care Surg 2017;83:19-24.
20. Khan S, Allard S, Weaver A, et al. A major haemorrhage protocol improves the delivery of blood component therapy and reduces waste in trauma massive transfusion. Injury 2013;44:587-92.
21. Pham HP, Shaz BH. Update on massive transfusion. Br J Anaesth 2013;111(Suppl 1):i71-82.
22. McDaniel LM, Neal MD, Sperry JL, et al. Use of a massive transfusion protocol in nontrauma patients: Activate away. J Am Coll Surg 2013;216:1103-9.
23. Martinez-Calle N, Hidalgo F, Alfonso A, et al. Implementation of a management protocol for massive bleeding reduces mortality in non-trauma patients: Results from a single centre audit. Med Intensiva 2016;40:550-9.
24. Borgman MA, Spinella PC, Perkins JG, et al. The ratio of blood products transfused affects mortality in patients receiving massive transfusions at a combat support hospital. J Trauma 2007;63:805-13.
25. Holcomb JB, del Junco DJ, Fox EE, et al. The prospective, observational, multicenter, major trauma transfusion (PROMMTT) study: Comparative effectiveness of a time-varying treatment with competing risks. JAMA Surg 2013;148:127-36.
26. Holcomb JB, Tilley BC, Baraniuk S, et al. Transfusion of plasma, platelets, and red blood cells in a 1:1:1 vs a 1:1:2 ratio and mortality in patients with severe trauma: The

PROPPR randomized clinical trial. JAMA 2015;313:471-82.
27. Mesar T, Larentzakis A, Dzik W, et al. Association between ratio of fresh frozen plasma to red blood cells during massive transfusion and survival among patients without traumatic injury. JAMA Surg 2017;152:574-80.
28. Etchill EW, Myers SP, McDaniel LM, et al. Should all massively transfused patients be treated equally? An analysis of massive transfusion ratios in the nontrauma setting. Crit Care Med 2017;45:1311-16.
29. Hanke AA, Horstmann H, Wilhelmi M. Point-of-care monitoring for the management of trauma-induced bleeding. Curr Opin Anaesthesiol 2017;30:250-6.
30. Einersen PM, Moore EE, Chapman MP, et al. Rapid thrombelastography thresholds for goal-directed resuscitation of patients at risk for massive transfusion. J Trauma Acute Care Surg 2017;82:114-19.
31. Da Luz LT, Nascimento B, Shankarakutty AK, et al. Effect of thromboelastography (TEG(R)) and rotational thromboelastometry (ROTEM(R)) on diagnosis of coagulopathy, transfusion guidance and mortality in trauma: Descriptive systematic review. Crit Care 2014;18:518.
32. Lier H, Vorweg M, Hanke A, Gorlinger K. Thromboelastometry guided therapy of severe bleeding. Essener Runde algorithm. Hamostaseologie 2013;33:51-61.
33. American College of Surgeons Trauma Quality Improvement Program. ACS-TQIP massive transfusion in trauma guidelines. Chicago: American College of Surgeons, 2013. [Available at https://www.facs.org/~/media/files/quality%20programs/trauma/tqip/massive%20transfusion%20in%20trauma%20guildelines.ashx (accessed July 22, 2017).]
34. Camazine MN, Hemmila MR, Leonard JC, et al. Massive transfusion policies at trauma centers participating in the American College of Surgeons Trauma Quality Improvement Program. J Trauma Acute Care Surg 2015;78:S48-53.

35. Yucel N, Lefering R, Maegele M, et al. Trauma Associated Severe Hemorrhage (TASH)-Score: Probability of mass transfusion as surrogate for life threatening hemorrhage after multiple trauma. J Trauma 2006;60:1228-36; discussion 36-7.
36. Cotton BA, Dossett LA, Haut ER, et al. Multicenter validation of a simplified score to predict massive transfusion in trauma. J Trauma 2010;69(Suppl 1):S33-9.
37. Rainer TH, Ho AM, Yeung JH, et al. Early risk stratification of patients with major trauma requiring massive blood transfusion. Resuscitation 2011;82:724-9.
38. McCluskey SA, Karkouti K, Wijeysundera DN, et al. Derivation of a risk index for the prediction of massive blood transfusion in liver transplantation. Liver Transpl 2006; 12:1584-93.
39. Karkouti K, O'Farrell R, Yau TM, et al. Prediction of massive blood transfusion in cardiac surgery. Can J Anaesth 2006;53:781-94.
40. Le Bas A, Chandraharan E, Addei A, Arulkumaran S. Use of the "obstetric shock index" as an adjunct in identifying significant blood loss in patients with massive postpartum hemorrhage. Int J Gynaecol Obstet 2014;124:253-5.
41. Boisen ML, Collins RA, Yazer MH, Waters JH. Pretransfusion testing and transfusion of uncrossmatched erythrocytes. Anesthesiology 2015;122:191-5.
42. Dutton RP, Shih D, Edelman BB, et al. Safety of uncrossmatched type-O red cells for resuscitation from hemorrhagic shock. J Trauma 2005;59:1445-9.
43. Goodell PP, Uhl L, Mohammed M, Powers AA. Risk of hemolytic transfusion reactions following emergency-release RBC transfusion. Am J Clin Pathol 2010;134:202-6.
44. Radkay L, Triulzi DJ, Yazer MH. Low risk of hemolysis after transfusion of uncrossmatched red blood cells. Immunohematology 2012;28:39-44.
45. Goodnough LT, Viele M, Fontaine MJ, et al. Implementation of a two-specimen requirement for verification of

ABO/Rh for blood transfusion. Transfusion 2009;49:1321-8.
46. Saverimuttu J, Greenfield T, Rotenko I, et al. Implications for urgent transfusion of uncrossmatched blood in the emergency department: The prevalence of clinically significant red cell antibodies within different patient groups. Emerg Med (Fremantle) 2003;15:239-43.
47. Strandenes G, Berseus O, Cap AP, et al. Low titer group O whole blood in emergency situations. Shock 2014;41 (Suppl 1):70-5.
48. Cid J, Lozano M, Ziman A, et al. Low frequency of anti-D alloimmunization following D+ platelet transfusion: The Anti-D Alloimmunization after D-incompatible Platelet Transfusions (ADAPT) study. Br J Haematol 2015; 168:598-603.
49. Gonzalez-Porras JR, Graciani IF, Perez-Simon JA, et al. Prospective evaluation of a transfusion policy of D+ red blood cells into D- patients. Transfusion 2008;48:1318-24.
50. Ooley PW, ed. Standards for blood banks and transfusion services. 30th ed. Bethesda, MD: AABB, 2016.
51. Agaronov M, DiBattista A, Christenson E, et al. Perception of low-titer group A plasma and potential barriers to using this product: A blood center's experience serving community and academic hospitals. Transfus Apher Sci 2016;55: 141-5.
52. Roback JD, Caldwell S, Carson J, et al. Evidence-based practice guidelines for plasma transfusion. Transfusion 2010;50:1227-39.
53. Backholer L, Green L, Huish S, et al. A paired comparison of thawed and liquid plasma. Transfusion 2017;57:881-9.
54. Spinella PC, Frazier E, Pidcoke HF, et al. All plasma products are not created equal: Characterizing differences between plasma products. J Trauma Acute Care Surg 2015; 78:S18-25.
55. Dudaryk R, Hess AS, Varon AJ, Hess JR. What is new in the blood bank for trauma resuscitation. Curr Opin Anaesthesiol 2015;28:206-9.

56. Wagner SJ. Whole blood and apheresis collections for blood components intended for transfusion. In: Fung MK, Eder AF, Spitalnik SL, Westhoff CM, eds. Technical manual. 19th ed. Bethesda, MD: AABB, 2017;6:125-60.
57. Dunbar NM, Yazer MH, for the BEST Collaborative. Safety of the use of group A plasma in trauma: The STAT study. Transfusion 2017 Jun 8. doi: 10.1111/trf.14139. [Epub ahead of print.]
58. Pidcoke HF, McFaul SJ, Ramasubramanian AK, et al. Primary hemostatic capacity of whole blood: A comprehensive analysis of pathogen reduction and refrigeration effects over time. Transfusion 2013;53(Suppl 1):137S-49S.
59. Jobes D, Wolfe Y, O'Neill D, et al. Toward a definition of "fresh" whole blood: An in vitro characterization of coagulation properties in refrigerated whole blood for transfusion. Transfusion 2011;51:43-51.
60. Reddoch KM, Pidcoke HF, Montgomery RK, et al. Hemostatic function of apheresis platelets stored at 4 degrees C and 22 degrees C. Shock 2014;41(Suppl 1):54-61.
61. Nair PM, Pidcoke HF, Cap AP, Ramasubramanian AK. Effect of cold storage on shear-induced platelet aggregation and clot strength. J Trauma Acute Care Surg 2014; 77:S88-93.
62. Yazer MH, Glackin EM, Triulzi DJ, et al. The effect of stationary versus rocked storage of whole blood on red blood cell damage and platelet function. Transfusion 2016;56: 596-604.
63. Seheult JN, Triulzi DJ, Alarcon LH, et al. Measurement of haemolysis markers following transfusion of uncrossmatched, low-titre, group O+ whole blood in civilian trauma patients: Initial experience at a level 1 trauma centre. Transfus Med 2017;27:30-5.
64. Wikkelsoe AJ, Afshari A, Stensballe J, et al. The FIB-PPH trial: Fibrinogen concentrate as initial treatment for postpartum haemorrhage: Study protocol for a randomised controlled trial. Trials 2012;13:110.

65. Rajan PV, Wing DA. Postpartum hemorrhage: Evidence-based medical interventions for prevention and treatment. Clin Obstet Gynecol 2010;53:165-81.
66. Collaborators WT. Effect of early tranexamic acid administration on mortality, hysterectomy, and other morbidities in women with post-partum haemorrhage (WOMAN): An international, randomised, double-blind, placebo-controlled trial. Lancet 2017;389:2105-16.
67. McCormack PL. Tranexamic acid: A review of its use in the treatment of hyperfibrinolysis. Drugs 2012;72:585-617.
68. Farrell NM, Wing HA, Burke PA, Huiras P. Addition of tranexamic acid to a traumatic injury massive transfusion protocol. Am J Health Syst Pharm 2015;72:1059-64.
69. Kashuk JL, Moore EE, Sawyer M, et al. Primary fibrinolysis is integral in the pathogenesis of the acute coagulopathy of trauma. Ann Surg 2010;252:434-42; discussion 43-4.
70. Roberts I, Shakur H, Coats T, et al. The CRASH-2 trial: A randomised controlled trial and economic evaluation of the effects of tranexamic acid on death, vascular occlusive events and transfusion requirement in bleeding trauma patients. Health Technol Assess 2013;17:1-79.
71. Franchini M, Mannucci PM. Adjunct agents for bleeding. Curr Opin Hematol 2014;21:503-8.
72. Desborough MJ, Oakland KA, Landoni G, et al. Desmopressin for treatment of platelet dysfunction and reversal of antiplatelet agents: A systematic review and meta-analysis of randomized controlled trials. J Thromb Haemost 2017;15:263-72.
73. Joseph B, Aziz H, Pandit V, et al. Prothrombin complex concentrate versus fresh-frozen plasma for reversal of coagulopathy of trauma: Is there a difference? World J Surg 2014;38:1875-81.
74. Levi M, Levy JH, Andersen HF, Truloff D. Safety of recombinant activated factor VII in randomized clinical trials. N Engl J Med 2010;363:1791-800.

75. Devlin R, Bonanno L, Badeaux J. The incidence of thromboembolism formation following the use of recombinant factor VIIa in patients suffering from blunt force trauma compared with penetrating trauma: A systematic review. JBI Database System Rev Implement Rep 2016;14:116-38.
76. Hauser CJ, Boffard K, Dutton R, et al. Results of the CONTROL trial: Efficacy and safety of recombinant activated Factor VII in the management of refractory traumatic hemorrhage. J Trauma 2010;69:489-500.
77. McQuilten ZK, Crighton G, Engelbrecht S, et al. Transfusion interventions in critical bleeding requiring massive transfusion: A systematic review. Transfus Med Rev 2015; 29:127-37.
78. Dutton RP, Parr M, Tortella BJ, et al. Recombinant activated factor VII safety in trauma patients: Results from the CONTROL trial. J Trauma 2011;71:12-19.
79. Lin Y, Moltzan CJ, Anderson DR, National Advisory Committee on Blood and Blood Products. The evidence for the use of recombinant factor VIIa in massive bleeding: Revision of the transfusion policy framework. Transfus Med 2012;22:383-94.

ADVERSE EFFECTS OF BLOOD TRANSFUSION

Because of the risk of adverse reactions, transfusion should be administered only when the benefits clearly outweigh the risks. Patients should be advised of the risks, benefits, and alternatives to transfusion and of the consequences of refusal of transfusion. Documentation of patient consent is required. All suspected transfusion reactions should be reported to the transfusion service for investigation and guidance on further recommendations for component therapy.

Acute Transfusion Reactions

Acute transfusion reactions occur during or within 24 hours after a transfusion. Most life-threatening transfusion reactions occur early in the course of transfusion; therefore, all patients should be monitored carefully throughout transfusion, and any adverse signs and symptoms should be investigated promptly. If a reaction occurs during the course of a multiple-unit transfusion, the unit currently being transfused may not necessarily be the cause of the reaction.

Acute Hemolytic Reactions

Hemolytic transfusion reactions (HTRs) are caused by immune-mediated lysis of incompatible red cells. Such reactions can be acute or delayed and can result in intravascular or extravascular hemolysis. An acute HTR (AHTR) occurs when incompatible red cells are transfused to a recipient who already has a clinically significant antibody to an antigen present on the transfused cells, as in the transfusion of group A red cells to a group O or group B recipient. Many fatal HTRs are the result of transfusion of ABO-incompatible blood; however, fatal HTRs caused by other blood group antibodies do occur. During fiscal years 2011 through 2015, more fatal HTRs caused by non-ABO blood group antibodies were reported to the Food and Drug Administration (FDA) than those caused by ABO incompatibility.[1]

Patient misidentification during patient sample collection, compatibility testing, or blood administration is the most common cause of ABO-incompatibility-induced acute hemolysis. Patients transfused at more than one health-care facility who develop non-ABO red cell antibodies can face increased risks because non-ABO antibodies identified at one facility may be unknown to other facilities. In one survey of patients in a health-care system who were known to have non-ABO antibodies, 64% had discrepancies in the records of the antibodies at more than one hospital.[2] AHTRs typically occur within minutes of the start of the infusion.

If the recipient's antibody fixes complement, as most often occurs with ABO-incompatible blood transfusions, an acute intravascular HTR results.[3] The anti-A and anti-B responsible are either immunoglobulin M (IgM) or complement-fixing immunoglobulin G (IgG). Complement fixation leads to pore formation and osmotic lysis. Water enters the cell through this pore, and osmotic intravascular lysis results, which produces hemoglobinemia. This can result in an increase of plasma hemoglobin to 200 mg/dL or more, which will lend plasma a pink to red color. If the plasma hemoglobin is only moderately increased, between 10 and 40 mg/dL, plasma discoloration may be less evident because of other pigments such as bilirubin (yellow) or methemalbumin (brown). The renal glomerulus filters free hemoglobin molecules once plasma haptoglobin is saturated; this results in hemoglobinuria.[4] These two signs are critical for recognition of an AHTR. Characteristic laboratory findings may also include failure to increase the hematocrit after transfusion, decreased haptoglobin, and increased lactate dehydrogenase (LDH). The direct antiglobulin test (DAT) can demonstrate complement or IgG, or may even be negative as a result of severe hemolysis. Serum bilirubin typically increases 6 to 12 hours later.

The severe clinical symptoms of shock and hypotension seen in an AHTR are caused by the generated complement fragments, anaphylatoxins C3a and C5a, and other mediators of inflammation.[3,4] In addition, hypotension can lead to renal ischemia, which may result in tubular necrosis and the development of acute renal failure. Hemoglobin scavenging of nitric oxide, a potent vasodilator, further promotes renal vasoconstriction, tubular necrosis, and renal failure.[5] The coagulation cascade may be activated as well, initiating disseminated intravascular coagulation (DIC). Clinical symptoms are in large part attributable to activation of the cytokine network, including the proinflammatory cytokines interleukin-1 (IL-1), IL-6, IL-8, and tumor necrosis factor-alpha (TNF-α), which produce fever, hypotension, and activation of white cells and the clotting cascade.[6,7]

The severity of an AHTR depends on the rate and amount of blood transfused. Generally, a larger volume of incompatible blood transfused and a faster infusion rate result in a more severe reaction. Treatment of an AHTR, a medical emergency, is described in Table 13. If any reaction is suspected, infusion of the unit should be stopped immediately, and additional Red Blood Cell (RBC) units should not be administered until the cause has been identified and corrected. Communication with the blood bank is critical. The occurrence of acute intravascular hemolysis in the absence of red cell incompatibility should prompt the search for a nonimmunologic cause of the hemolysis (see below). Whereas most AHTRs are intravascular, if the antibody does not fix complement or fixes only to C3, the resulting reaction will be an acute extravascular HTR (Table 14). Acute extravascular HTRs are not associated with the serious clinical symptom complex seen in acute intravascular HTRs, because extravascular HTRs involve much less generation of proinflammatory cytokines.[9] Acute extravascular HTRs typically present with fever, a

Table 13. Workup of an Acute Transfusion Reaction

If an acute transfusion reaction occurs:
1. Stop blood component transfusion immediately.
2. Verify that the correct unit was given to the correct patient.
3. Maintain IV access and ensure adequate urine output with an appropriate crystalloid or colloid solution.
4. Maintain blood pressure and pulse.
5. Maintain adequate ventilation.
6. Notify attending physician and blood bank.
7. Obtain blood/urine for transfusion reaction workup.
8. Send report of reaction, samples, blood bag, and administration set to blood bank.
9. Blood bank performs workup of suspected transfusion reaction as follows:
    A. A clerical check is performed to ensure that the right blood component was transfused to the right patient.
    B. The plasma is visually evaluated for hemoglobinemia.
    C. A direct antiglobulin test is performed.
    D. Other serologic testing is repeated as needed (ABO, Rh, crossmatch).

If an intravascular hemolytic reaction is confirmed:
1. Monitor renal status (BUN, creatinine).
2. Initiate diuresis; avoid fluid overload if renal failure is present.
3. Analyze urine for hemoglobinuria.
4. Monitor coagulation status (PT, aPTT, fibrinogen, platelet count).
5. Monitor for signs of hemolysis (LDH, bilirubin, haptoglobin, plasma hemoglobin).
6. Monitor hemoglobin and hematocrit.
7. Repeat compatibility testing (crossmatch).
8. **Consult with blood bank physician before further transfusion.**

If bacterial contamination is suspected:
1. Obtain blood culture of patient.

Table 13. Workup of an Acute Transfusion Reaction (Continued)

2. Return unit or empty blood bag to blood bank for culture and Gram stain.
3. Maintain circulation and urine output.
4. Initiate broad-spectrum antibiotic treatment as appropriate; revise antibiotic regimen on the basis of microbiologic results.
5. Monitor for signs of DIC, renal failure, and respiratory failure.

Adapted from Wu Y, Mantha S, Snyder EL. Transfusion reactions. In: Hoffman R, Benz EF Jr, Shattil SJ, et al, eds. Hematology: Basic principles and practice. 5th ed. New York: Churchill Livingstone, 2008:2267-75.
IV = intravenous; BUN = blood urea nitrogen; PT = prothrombin time; aPTT = activated partial thromboplastin time; LDH = lactate dehydrogenase; DIC = disseminated intravascular coagulation.

positive DAT caused by antibody binding to the transfused incompatible red cells, and a decreasing hematocrit without any overt signs of bleeding. Hemoglobinemia and hemoglobinuria are rarely seen. Severe hemolytic reactions may also occur in association with the infusion of incompatible plasma, which may occur with transfusion of ABO-incompatible platelets (such as group O platelets to a group A patient) and, rarely, with infusion of intravenous immune globulin (IVIG) or intermediate-purity Factor VIII concentrates.[10-12]

Sickle Cell Hemolytic Transfusion Reaction Syndrome

Multitransfused patients with sickle cell disease have a greater incidence of red cell alloimmunization because of frequent transfusion and red cell phenotype differences from the general donor population. HTRs in sickle cell disease can precipitate a hemolytic crisis and result in a greater degree of anemia than before transfusion because of bystander hemolysis of autologous red cells and/or the sickle cell HTR syndrome.[13,14] In this syndrome, there is a suppression of endogenous erythropoiesis and a

Table 14. Acute Transfusion Reactions[8]

Type	Incidence	Signs and Symptoms	Usual Cause	Treatment	Prevention
Intravascular hemolytic (immune)	ABO/Rh mismatch: 1:40,000 AHTR: 1:76,000 Fatal HTR: 1:1.8 million	Hemoglobinemia and hemoglobinuria, fever, chills, anxiety, shock, DIC, dyspnea, chest pain, flank pain, oliguria	ABO incompatibility (clerical error) or other complement-fixing red cell antibody	Stop transfusion; hydrate, support blood pressure and respiration; induce diuresis; treat shock and DIC, if present	Ensure proper sample and recipient identification
Extravascular hemolytic (immune)	1:100 RBC transfusions	Fever, malaise, indirect hyperbilirubinemia, increased LDH, urine urobilinogen, decreasing hematocrit	IgG non-complement-fixing antibody	Monitor hematocrit, renal and hepatic function, coagulation profile; no acute treatment generally required	Review historical records; ensure proper sample and recipient identification; give antigen-negative units as appropriate; possible high-dose IVIG

Reaction	Frequency	Signs/Symptoms	Etiology	Management	Prevention
Febrile	0.1% to 1% with universal leukocyte reduction	Fever, chills	Antibodies to leukocytes or plasma proteins; hemolysis; passive cytokine infusion; bacterial contamination; commonly due to patient's underlying condition	Stop transfusion; give antipyretics, eg, acetaminophen; for rigors in adults, use meperidine 25 to 50 mg IV or IM	Pretransfusion antipyretic for recurrences; leukocyte-reduced blood components
Allergic (mild to severe)	1:100 to 1:33	Urticaria (hives), dyspnea, wheezing, throat tightening; rarely, hypotension or anaphylaxis	Antibodies to plasma proteins; rarely, antibodies to IgA	Stop transfusion; give antihistamine (PO or IM); if severe, epinephrine and/or steroids	Pretransfusion antihistamine for recurrences; washed red cells, if recurrent or severe; check pretransfusion IgA levels in patients with a history of anaphylaxis to transfusion

(Continued)

Table 14. Acute Transfusion Reactions[a] (Continued)

Type	Incidence	Signs and Symptoms	Usual Cause	Treatment	Prevention
Transfusion-associated circulatory overload (TACO)	1%	Dyspnea, hypertension, pulmonary edema, cardiac arrhythmias	Too rapid and/or excessive blood transfusion volume	Induce diuresis; phlebotomy; support cardiorespiratory system as needed	Avoid rapid or excessive transfusion volume
Transfusion-related acute lung injury (TRALI)	1:1200 to 1:190,000	Dyspnea, fever, hypoxia, pulmonary edema, hypotension, normal pulmonary capillary wedge pressure	Donor HLA or leukocyte antibody transfused with plasma in component; neutrophil-priming lipid mediator; less commonly, recipient antibody to donor white cells	Support blood pressure and respiration (may require intubation)	Notify transfusion service and blood center to test donor(s); quarantine remaining components from donor(s)

Hypotension	Depends on clinical setting	Hypotension, tachycardia	Bradykinin generation; may be exacerbated by ACE inhibitor	Stop transfusion; give fluids; use Trendelenberg position	Discontinue ACE inhibitor; slower transfusion rate
Bacterial contamination	Varies by component	Rigors, chills, fever, shock	Contaminated blood component	Stop transfusion; support blood pressure; culture patient and blood unit; give antibiotics; notify blood transfusion service	Care in donor selection, blood collection and storage; careful attention to arm preparation for phlebotomy

AHTR = acute hemolytic transfusion reaction; DIC = disseminated intravascular coagulation; RBC = Red Blood Cell; LDH = lactate dehydrogenase; IgG = immunoglobulin G; IVIG = intravenous immune globulin; IV = intravenous; IM = intramuscular; PO = by mouth; ACE = angiotensin-converting enzyme.

decrease in the absolute number of hemoglobin-S-containing red cells.[13,14] Painful crisis in a patient with sickle cell disease after transfusion should suggest the occurrence of sickle cell HTR syndrome. Further transfusion in the setting of bystander hemolysis or sickle cell HTR syndrome may exacerbate the anemia and may even prove fatal. Therefore, the decision to transfuse RBCs must be carefully measured with consideration given to the fact that not transfusing may be most prudent. Iatrogenic blood loss should be avoided. To avoid additional transfusion in this setting, corticosteroids and erythropoietin are often administered, as is IVIG.[15,16] Serologic studies may not provide a clear explanation for HTRs in these patients, in part because the presence of multiple alloantibodies may make the serologic diagnosis difficult. On the other hand, alloantibodies may not be detected at all; in these patients, the mechanism may be related to the induction of phosphatidylserine exposure on donor red cells, which leads to accelerated donor red cell destruction that eventually leads to autologous red cell destruction as well.[17]

Drug-Induced Hemolysis

Many drugs can induce the production of antibodies against red cells and cause hemolysis. Although drug-induced hemolysis is not a transfusion reaction, it can be readily confused with an HTR in the transfused patient. In drug-induced hemolysis, both autologous and transfused red cells will be eliminated. Typically, there is a positive DAT result, and the serum will react with red cells in the presence, but not the absence, of the offending drug. Clinically, drug-induced hemolysis may be indistinguishable from an HTR. The hemolysis may be severe and even fatal. Laboratory evaluation requires referral to a specialized laboratory, and results can be delayed. Therefore, treatment consists of discontinuing the drug, providing supportive care, and administering transfusion to maintain adequate oxygen-carrying capacity. Cefotetan and ceftriaxone are among the most common causes of drug-induced hemolysis; however, nonsteroidal anti-inflammatory drugs should not be overlooked.[18]

Nonimmune Hemolysis

Mechanical hemolysis of transfused blood, caused by shear stress imposed on erythrocytes, can occur with artificial heart valves, with extracorporeal circulation, or with transfusion through small-bore catheters under high pressure. Administration of hypotonic saline solutions, 5% dextrose in water, distilled water, or certain medications in the same line as the blood infusion can result in osmotic lysis of transfused red cells. Heating above 42 C that results from a malfunction of the blood warmer, or freezing because of exposure to ice or a refrigerator malfunction, may hemolyze blood before transfusion. Hemoglobinuria may occur in nonimmune hemolysis. Transfusion of hemolyzed blood can cause hyperkalemia and transient renal impairment. Other causes of acute hemolysis such as certain bacterial infections[19] may also need to be ruled out. The cause of hemoglobinemia and/or hemoglobinuria must be evaluated by a transfusion medicine physician as soon as possible, because delay in the recognition of an immune HTR could lead to serious clinical complications.

Febrile Nonhemolytic Transfusion Reactions

Fever is a common sign of a transfusion reaction (Table 14) and may be the first sign of a reaction. Fever results from the production of pyrogens (IL-1, IL-6, and TNF-α) that act on the thermoregulatory center in the hypothalamus through the intermediary of prostaglandin E2. Fever may be caused by the patient's underlying condition; thus fever, per se, is not a contraindication for administering a blood transfusion. A febrile nonhemolytic transfusion reaction (FNHTR) is defined as occurring during or within 4 hours of transfusion and involving either a fever greater than 38 C orally and a change of ≥ 1 C from the pretransfusion temperature, or chills and/or rigors. An FNHTR may occur without a measured fever if chills/rigors are the only presenting symptoms. Febrile reactions may be attributed to antibodies directed against transfused leukocytes or platelets. The resulting antigen-antibody reactions trigger phagocytes to release endogenous pyrogens, an action which causes fever.[6,19] Alternatively, leukocytes in cellular blood components may produce pyrogens during storage.[20] The use of leukocyte-reduced blood components can mitigate, but not necessarily eliminate, these reactions.[21,22]

Most FNHTRs respond to treatment with antipyretics. In general, aspirin should not be used in thrombocytopenic patients. For such patients, acetaminophen or nonsteroidal anti-inflammatory agents are preferred. Acetaminophen has commonly been prescribed for prophylaxis; however, the evidence supporting efficacy of this practice is questionable.[23] FNHTRs are rarely serious, but rigors can be a significant stress for a patient with compromised cardiorespiratory status. Rigors may be treated with opioids, although such drugs should be used with caution in patients with impaired respiratory drive. Antihistamines do not prevent febrile reactions and have no role in prophylaxis or treatment of febrile reactions.

Allergic Reactions

The estimated incidence of allergic reactions depends upon the component, and ranges from 2% of platelet transfusions to 0.1% to 0.5% of RBC transfusions.[24] Allergic reactions are most commonly mild with localized pruritus and urticaria. However they can exhibit a spectrum of severity up to angioedema, bronchospasm, and hypotension, seen in less than 10%. Some patients appear more susceptible than others.[25,26]

Platelets stored in platelet additive solution, which requires reduction of donor plasma and replacement with the additive solution, have a lower rate of allergic reactions.[27] (See Chapter 1: Blood Components.) Because allergic reactions are so common, diphenhydramine is often ordered as prophylactic premedication. However, in a prospective randomized study, this practice was not shown to decrease the rate of urticarial reactions.[28] Leukocyte reduction of components does not prevent allergic reactions.

Anaphylactic reactions can be caused by antibodies to IgA, haptoglobin, or C4 (Chido/Rodgers blood group antigens).[29,30]

For severe allergic or anaphylactic reactions, the transfusion should be stopped immediately, and intravenous (IV) access should be secured while fluid resuscitation and treatment with epinephrine and/or steroids are started. Severe reactions may require treatment with vasopressors and intubation. When further transfusion is indicated, washed cellular blood components or plasma-reduced platelets should be considered.[31] Transfusion of plasma and cryoprecipitate to such patients presents a difficult problem that requires a careful risk/benefit analysis. Pretransfusion treatment with high-dose corticosteroids, antihistamines, or H2 blockers should be considered, and the immediate availability of epinephrine should be ensured. A typical dose schedule is to medicate the patient 30 to 60 minutes before transfusion with 100 mg of IV hydrocortisone and 25 to 50 mg of diphenhydramine given orally or parenterally. Severely IgA-deficient patients who have made anti-IgA may require IgA-deficient plasma, which can be obtained through rare-donor registries.

Transfusion-Associated Circulatory Overload

Transfusion-associated circulatory overload (TACO) develops when the patient is unable to compensate for a fluid challenge in the setting of transfusion. Signs and symptoms of TACO include headache, cough, shortness of breath, congestion of pulmonary vasculature, increased central venous pressure, congestive heart failure, and systolic hypertension (>50 mm Hg increase). A review of hospital hemovigilance data found a significant proportion (32%) of TACO cases associated with new onset fever.[32] Brain natriuretic peptide (BNP) can be useful in distinguishing TACO from other causes of respiratory distress. Symptoms usually subside if the transfusion is stopped and the patient is placed in a sitting position and given oxygen and diuretics to remove fluid. (If symptoms persist, phlebotomy may be necessary.[33]) Rarely, hypertension with volume overload can lead to flash pulmonary edema. To avoid hypervolemia, blood components should not be infused at a rate faster than 2 to 4 mL/kg/hour. Slower rates are needed for patients at risk for TACO, such as patients with chronic anemia who have an expanded plasma volume or patients with compromised cardiac and/or pulmonary function. In these situations, a single or split unit of blood can be transfused slowly over time, in a period not to exceed 4 hours. TACO has become recognized as the second most common cause of transfusion-associated fatalities.[1]

Transfusion-Related Acute Lung Injury

Dyspnea, fever, chills, hypotension, and new-onset bilateral pulmonary edema associated with transfusion may indicate transfusion-related acute lung injury (TRALI). TRALI has been defined as acute lung injury with hypoxemia and PaO_2/FiO_2 ≤300 or SpO_2 <90% on room air, when no prior risk factors for acute lung injury existed before transfusion, with the onset of symptoms within 6 hours of transfusion.[34] It is differentiated from TACO by the lack of left atrial hypertension, nonelevated BNP levels, and unresponsiveness to diuresis.[34,35]

The infusion of HLA- or granulocyte-specific antibody in plasma-containing components, and the antibody being reactive with a recipient antigen, is hypothesized as the most common cause of this reaction. The donor of the implicated unit is often a multiparous woman.[36] Less commonly, recipient antibodies directed against donor leukocytes are implicated as a cause of TRALI. Alternatively, oxidation of membrane lipids produced by donor leukocytes during storage may prime recipient neutrophils so that a second stimulus, such as inflammation, infection, or tissue injury, results in the release of vasoactive mediators (the two-hit hypothesis).[37] Recipient factors may also determine susceptibility to TRALI because, in look-back cases, not all recipients of blood from an implicated donor manifest TRALI, even when there is HLA antigen-antibody concordance.[38,39] Neutrophil extracellular traps (NETs), composed of decondensed chromatin decorated with granular proteins, whose formation requires activation and release of neutrophil DNA, have been identified in the lungs and plasma in TRALI patients, pointing to the importance of platelet-neutrophil interaction in the pathophysiology of TRALI.[40]

In its full form, TRALI presents most commonly within 2 to 6 hours of a transfusion as marked respiratory distress, hypoxia, hypotension, fever, and bilateral pulmonary edema.[34,35] However, milder forms of TRALI may be difficult to recognize. TRALI reactions typically resolve within 48 to 72 hours, although the mortality rate is approximately 10%. In most instances, no special requirements are necessary to manage further transfusions; however, leukocyte-reduced components are indicated for subsequent transfusions if the reaction was caused by recipient HLA antibodies. The treatment of TRALI reactions is supportive. The patient may require supplemental oxygen, endotracheal intubation, and respiratory support until the intra-alveolar fluid can be resorbed. Diuresis is not indicated. The role of steroids in therapy is not clear. Fluid support may be necessary for resuscitation in the event of hypotension and marked movement of fluid from plasma to the extravascular space.

Suspected TRALI reactions should be reported to the blood bank immediately to ascertain information about the donor(s) of the transfused blood components and to allow the quarantine or recall of additional components from the donor(s). A test for HLA and granulocyte antibodies in donor plasma—and, if that test is positive, HLA and granulocyte antigen typing of the recipient—may help establish the diagnosis. Because TRALI is the most common cause of transfusion-associated mortality in the United States and fatal reactions have been linked to components produced from multiparous female donors, virtually all US blood suppliers are no longer producing plasma from these donors in order to decrease the risk of TRALI.[41] Additionally, many blood collectors are now also screening apheresis platelet donors for HLA antibodies.

Hypotensive Reactions to Transfusion

Hypotensive reactions following platelet and red cell transfusions have been reported.[42-44] These reactions are defined as a decrease in systolic blood pressure of ≥30 mm Hg and systolic blood pressure ≤80 mm Hg in adults, and in infants or children, a decrease of >25% from the baseline systolic blood pressure. To be considered transfusion-associated, the hypotension should occur during or within 1 hour of transfusion, and it may also be seen with facial flushing, dyspnea, or abdominal cramps. However, in most cases, hypotension is the sole manifestation. These reactions appear to involve the generation of bradykinin from activation of the kinin pathway, caused by contact of plasma with artificial surfaces. Patients on extracorporeal circulation and angiotensin-converting enzyme (ACE) inhibitors may be at increased risk. (See Chapter 8: Therapeutic Apheresis.) Transfusion-associated hypotension typically resolves within minutes of the cessation of the transfusion. Whenever such reactions occur, they must be differentiated from vasovagal reactions, TRALI, HTRs, bacterial contamination, anaphylaxis, and the patient's underlying medical condition. This is best accomplished by reporting these reactions to the transfusion service for investigation.

Bacterial Contamination

Bacterial contamination of stored blood poses a rare but serious risk to the transfusion recipient. Bacteria can enter a blood bag because of improper preparation of the skin at the venipuncture site at the time of phlebotomy or during component preparation or handling, or because of occult bacteremia in the donor. The overall rate of bacterial contamination of blood collections determined by prospective culture has been reported to be as high as 0.3%, although the incidence of serious clinically recognized reactions is much lower. Skin flora (ie, *Staphylococcus* and *Propionibacterium*) are the most common isolates from prospectively cultured units, but other species are more often implicated in clinical reactions. Gram-negative rods (ie, *Acinetobacter*, *Klebsiella*, and *Escherichia*) are more common than gram-positive cocci (ie, *Staphylococcus* and *Streptococcus*) in fatal reactions to contaminated RBC and platelet units.[45,46] Bacteria such as *Yersinia* or *Pseudomonas,* which are capable of growing at low temperatures in an iron-rich environment, may proliferate in RBC units. Although contaminated RBC units may appear dark or contain clots, visual inspection of components is not sensitive for detection of bacterial contamination.

During or after the transfusion, the patient may develop rigors, high fever, dyspnea, hypotension, and shock. Hemoglobinemia and hemoglobinuria are usually absent, and the posttransfusion DAT is usually negative. It is essential that any transfusion in progress be stopped when a contaminated unit is suspected. Aggressive resuscitative therapy and broad-spectrum antibiotics should be started immediately when a septic transfusion reaction is suspected. Additional components from the same donation, a common possibility with split apheresis components, could be infected and must be recalled. Therefore, suspected septic transfusion reactions should be reported immediately to the transfusion service and in turn to the blood collection center in order to prevent similar or even more severe reactions in other recipients.

The suspected unit should be evaluated by the microbiology laboratory, and blood cultures should also be drawn from the patient. Septic reactions may not manifest until several hours after the transfusion of a unit of contaminated blood. Adoption of methods to limit and detect bacterial contamination in platelet components[47,48] have decreased but not eliminated septic transfusion reactions. A study of more than 1 million apheresis platelet donations prospectively screened by culture found 186 donations with positive cultures; transfusion of all but one such donation was prevented. Components that screened negative were still implicated in 20 septic reactions, including three fatalities.[49]

Thermal Effects

The rapid transfusion of blood directly from refrigerator storage can result in hypothermia and consequent cardiac arrythmia or arrest. Conversely, overwarming blood can produce hemolysis. Blood should be warmed only by using an FDA-approved blood-warming device. (See Chapter 4: Transfusion Practices.) Warming blood with heating pads, hot tap water, or in a microwave oven is unacceptable.

Metabolic Complications

Blood is anticoagulated with citrate, which chelates calcium ions. If citrated blood is infused rapidly and the ionized calcium level decreases transiently, the patient may complain of tingling around the mouth (circumoral paresthesia) and in the fingers.[50] These symptoms subside quickly if the transfusion is slowed, because citrate is rapidly metabolized by patients with normal liver function. Under no circumstances should calcium be added to a unit of blood, because it could reverse the anticoagulant effect of the citrate, resulting in large blood clots.

During storage of RBC units, there is reversible leakage of potassium into the supernatant. Although the potassium concentration may be high, the total amount of potassium in an RBC unit is usually inconsequential. Hyperkalemia caused by the massive infusion of stored blood is rare. Hyperkalemia may be a concern in neonates (especially in the context of exchange transfusion) and sometimes in liver transplantation, pediatric cardiac surgery, and renal failure. Washing of red cells, removal of the supernatant, or use of blood less than 7 days old can be helpful in such cases. If irradiation is required, it may be best to wash after irradiation is performed.[50] With large-volume transfusion, the production of bicarbonate from the infused citrate more often produces an alkalosis, which results in hypokalemia that may require potassium administration.[51]

Delayed Hemolytic Transfusion Reactions

Delayed HTRs (DHTRs) occur when the survival of transfused red cells is decreased after production of an alloantibody response in a recipient days or weeks after the transfusion episode. The difference in the time of antibody production relates to whether it is an anamnestic response (days) or a primary response (weeks) to transfusion. It has been estimated that, with each additional unit of blood transfused, there is a 2% to 6% risk of immunizing a recipient to a red cell antigen other than the RhD antigen.[52] Most DHTRs are extravascular, and they are often associated with antibodies to Rh and Kell system antigens. Because the antibodies involved in extravascular DHTRs rarely fix complement, the clinical signs and symptoms are usually much less severe than are those associated with intravascular AHTRs. IgG-mediated phagocytosis results in inflammatory cytokine production but at a lower level than in AHTRs.[9] Because of the low level of inflammatory response and the lack of complement activation, patients with DHTRs often manifest only slight fever, weakness, and symptoms referable to anemia. A positive DAT result will be caused by the coating of the transfused donor red cells with recipient antibody. Destruction of the transfused red cells may cause anemia and indirect hyperbilirubinemia. Other laboratory findings may include an elevated reticulocyte count, increased LDH, and decreased haptoglobin. Hemoglobinemia is unusual. In the rare situations when transfusion is necessary but compatible blood is not obtainable, high-dose IVIG given before transfusion may prevent a DHTR.[53]

Intravascular DHTRs also occur and often are associated with antibodies to the Duffy (Fy^a or Fy^b) or Kidd (Jk^a or Jk^b) blood group system antigens. The C5b-9 component of complement may be fixed to the red cell membrane, and hemolysis with hemoglobinemia and hemoglobinuria may occur. However, the rate of generation of C3a, C5a, proinflammatory cytokines, and other biologic response modifiers is lower than in an intravascular AHTR; thus, the clinical symptoms in a DHTR are rarely life threatening. If a patient shows signs of a severe transfusion reaction, however, treatment should follow that described for an intravascular AHTR. DHTRs are also observed in ABO- and Rh-mismatched hematopoietic cell and solid organ transplantations.

Posttransfusion Purpura

Posttransfusion purpura (PTP) is characterized by the onset of profound thrombocytopenia 1 to 3 weeks after transfusion. All types of blood components have been implicated in PTP. In these reactions, there is an antibody response to a platelet antigen. Most cases have been associated with antibodies to human platelet antigen (HPA)-1a on the glycoprotein IIb/IIIa complex, but other platelet antigens have also been implicated. The diagnosis is established by the finding of a platelet-specific antibody in an antigen-negative patient. The thrombocytopenia of PTP typically persists for 2 to 3 weeks and resolves spontaneously, without treatment. The most likely pathophysiologic explanation for PTP is that, early in the course of an alloimmune response, the patient produces low-affinity antibodies that cross-react with autologous platelets. As the immune response naturally matures, low-affinity cross-reacting clones are eliminated and a pure alloantibody remains. The treatment of PTP is dependent on the clinical picture. Stable patients with low risk for hemorrhage may be followed closely until the platelet count returns to normal. Patients with significant bleeding or risk for hemorrhage should receive treatment to shorten the course of thrombocytopenia. High-dose IVIG has been reported to abruptly increase the platelet count.[54] Rarely, plasma exchange has been tried to remove the causative antibody.[55] (See Chapter 8: Therapeutic Apheresis.) Platelet transfusion is indicated for severe bleeding, but prophylactic platelet transfusion is futile and may delay recovery. There is no utility in transfusing antigen-negative platelets, even when a specificity is identified, because that patient is destroying perfectly matched autologous platelets. Steroids have not been shown to shorten the course of PTP.

Graft-vs-Host Disease

Graft-vs-host disease (GVHD), a well-recognized complication of allogeneic hematopoietic cell transplantation, can also occur after the transfusion of immunocompetent donor lymphocytes, usually to an immunoincompetent recipient.[56,57] Transfusion-associated GVHD (TA-GVHD) has also been observed after the transfusion of cellular components from HLA-homozygous donors to immunocompetent recipients who are heterozygous for the HLA haplotype.[58] Although the latter occurs more frequently after transfusion of blood from first- or second-degree relatives, it has been reported to occur also with the transfusion of blood from unrelated HLA-homozygous donors.[59]

GVHD is initiated by alloreactive donor T-cell recognition of host histocompatibility antigens.[60] Donor lymphocytes engraft in the recipient, proliferate, and attack host tissue. TA-GVHD typically begins 10 to 12 days after transfusion and is characterized by fever, skin rash, diarrhea, hepatitis, and marrow aplasia. TA-GVHD is fatal in most cases, usually because of host marrow failure that results in overwhelming infection or bleeding. TA-GVHD can be prevented by x-ray or gamma irradiation, or pathogen inactivation of cellular blood components, which renders donor lymphocytes incapable of proliferating.[61] (See Chapter 1: Blood Components.) In addition, all HLA-matched components and all cellular components from blood relatives should be irradiated, regardless of patient diagnosis.

Hemosiderosis

One mL of red cells contains 1 mg of iron. Therefore, an RBC unit may contain 150 to 250 mg of iron. In persons with chronic anemia, the continued need for red cell transfusion results in the accumulation of iron, which can eventually produce organ damage, particularly in the heart, liver, and pancreatic islets. In chronically transfused patients, treatment with iron chelation therapy is usually begun after 10 to 20 transfusions.[62] There is no physiologic mechanism for the excretion of excess iron. The parenteral iron chelator deferoxamine can prevent the complications of iron overload in patients undergoing chronic red cell transfusion therapy,[63] but it has a high rate of noncompliance. Better compliance may be achieved with deferasirox. Deferasirox is a daily oral iron chelator that is approved in the United States for treatment of transfusional iron overload in patients older than

2 years of age.[64] Red cell exchange by apheresis has also been used to limit iron accumulation in patients with sickle cell disease who require repeated transfusions. (See Chapter 8: Therapeutic Apheresis.)

Air Embolism

Air embolism is rarely a problem with conventional transfusion techniques. Rapid infusion devices can infuse as much as 200 mL of air in 4 seconds. Air embolism may also be seen with the use of intraoperative blood recovery. The frequency of fatal air embolism after the infusion of recovered blood is 1:30,000 to 1:38,000.[65] Air embolism produces acute cardiopulmonary insufficiency, because the air tends to migrate to the right ventricle, where it produces outlet obstruction. Acute cyanosis, pain, cough, arrythmia, shock, and cardiac arrest may result. Patients with a patent foramen ovale may also present with central nervous system symptoms. Immediate treatment includes placing the patient head-down on the left side in an attempt to dislodge the air bubble from the pulmonary valve.

Transfusion-Transmitted Diseases

Allogeneic blood donations are tested for the presence of hepatitis B surface antigen (HBsAg); antibody to hepatitis B core antigen (anti-HBc); antibody to hepatitis C virus (anti-HCV); antibody to human immunodeficiency virus, types 1 and 2 (anti-HIV-1/2); antibody to human T-cell lymphotropic virus, types I and II (anti-HTLV-I/II); and antibody to *Trypanosoma cruzi* (Chagas disease); as well as undergoing a serologic test for syphilis and nucleic acid amplification testing (NAT) for hepatitis B virus (HBV), HCV, HIV, Zika virus (ZIKV), and West Nile virus (WNV). In areas where *Babesia* is endemic, serologic testing of donors for *Babesia* is common. Despite extensive donor screening and testing, infections can still be transmitted by blood transfusion.[66] (See Table 15.)

Table 15. Residual Risk of Transfusion-Transmitted Infectious Diseases[66]

	Residual Risk per Donated Unit	Window Period (days)
HIV	1:1,467,000	9.1
HCV	1:1,149,000	7.4
HBV	1:843,000 to 1:1,208,000	26.5 to 18.5

HIV = human immunodeficiency virus; HCV = hepatitis C virus; HBV = hepatitis B virus

Hepatitis

HCV accounts for most posttransfusion hepatitis. Almost all cases of posttransfusion HCV were acquired before the implementation of donor serologic screening in 1990. Less than 20% of acute infections are symptomatic, and 85% of infections become chronic, but they are usually asymptomatic. In contrast to HCV, acute HBV infection is symptomatic in 30% to 50% of adults but in less than 10% of children younger than 5 years of age. Recent estimates of the window period for HBV and HCV are 26.5 to 18.5 days for HBV and 7 days for HCV. Estimates of the per-unit risk of transfusion-transmitted hepatitis are 1:843,000 to 1:1,208,000 for HBV and approximately 1 in 1.1 million for HCV.[66] Testing for HBV by NAT found a positivity rate of 1 in 410,540 donations.[67] Hepatitis A transmission has occurred with plasma derivatives but is not a substantial risk for blood components. Hepatitis E virus (HEV) caused 26 cases of clinical hepatitis documented by the Centers for Disease Control and Prevention (CDC) between 2005 and 2012. HEV infection occurs among adults and is usually asymptomatic, with a seroprevalence in healthy individuals of 6.25% in Western Europe, North America, and Japan. Transmission by transfusion has been reported in Japan. Testing for infection is available only from reference laboratories.[68]

HIV

Transfusion-transmitted HIV has declined markedly since the implementation of antibody testing in 1985. The clinical manifestations of transfusion-transmitted HIV infection are similar to those of infections acquired through other routes. Currently, transmission by transfusion is very rare. The current estimated window period for HIV is 9 days. The per-unit risk of HIV transmission is estimated to be approximately 1 in 1.5 million in the United States.[66]

West Nile Virus

WNV, a mosquito-borne virus primarily infecting birds, has infected humans as incidental hosts and thus has become a major public health concern in North America. Since 1999, WNV has caused several thousand cases of febrile illness and neuroinvasive disease such as encephalitis, meningitis, and spastic paralysis. WNV infections occur during the spring and summer months, when mosquitoes are active. Evidence of transmission through transfusion, breastfeeding, and organ transplantation has been reported.[69,70] WNV NAT has been performed throughout the United States since 2003, and it has prevented many cases of potential transmission. However, the low levels of viremia in infected blood donors, especially during the early stages of infection, have required complex seasonal and temporal testing algorithms using pooled and individual donor samples.

Zika

Zika virus is an enveloped RNA flavivirus. An outbreak was noted in Brazil in early 2015 with rapid spread throughout the Americas over the next year. The most common symptoms of infection include transient low-grade fever, itchy maculopapular rash, arthritis or arthralgia, and nonpurulent conjunctivitis. However, approximately 80% of infected individuals are asymptomatic. Infection has been associated with Guillan-Barré syndrome, and microcephaly in infants born to women infected during pregnancy.[71]

The *Aedes aegypti* mosquito is its most common vector in the Americas, but ZIKV can also be sexually transmitted. Probable transmission of ZIKV by blood transfusion has been reported.[72]

The FDA issued revised guidance in August 2016 requiring testing of all US blood donors for ZIKV using individual donation (ID)-NAT under an approved investigational new device application. Alternatively, use of pathogen inactivation technology for platelets and plasma using an FDA-approved pathogen inactivation device could be substituted for ZIKV testing. Chikungunya and dengue, two additional emerging transfusion-transmitted infectious diseases, are also susceptible to pathogen inactivation.

Other Viruses

Cytomegalovirus (CMV) infection is a major concern in immunosuppressed recipients. Latent CMV infection is common among blood donors. CMV DNA can be found in the leukocytes of seropositive and seronegative donors.[73] Transmission of CMV can be significantly reduced with equivalent efficacy by the use of either seronegative or leukocyte-reduced blood components.[73,74] Pathogen inactivation also produces a component with a reduced risk of CMV transmission.

HTLVs are retroviruses unrelated to HIV. They are causally associated with adult T-cell lymphoma-leukemia and peripheral neuropathy (HTLV-associated myelopathy). HTLV-I/II infections are rare in the United States. Because these viruses are strongly associated with white cells, leukocyte reduction may further reduce their transmission by transfusion.

Parvovirus B19 causes erythema infectiosum in childhood. This virus can infect red cell precursors in marrow, and, in patients with accelerated hematopoiesis, it can cause hypoplastic or aplastic anemia. Parvovirus can cause aplastic crisis in sickle cell disease, nonimmune hydrops if acquired in pregnancy, and marrow transplant failure. Parvovirus B19 is common in the general population. Transmission by blood transfusion occurs but seldom causes significant disease.[75]

Epstein-Barr virus and human herpesvirus 8 are transmissible by transfusion, but they do not appear to be of clinical significance in transfusion recipients.

Parasite-Related Disease

Babesia is the most common transfusion-transmitted parasite in the United States, with 11 deaths from babesiosis reported to the FDA between 2005 and 2010. The parasitic reservoir is distributed in the eastern and north-central United States. Available serologic tests are inadequate for blood donor screening, but tests for blood donors are currently in development.[76]

Transfusion-transmitted malaria is uncommon in the United States, but it does occur.[77] The most frequently implicated species is *Plasmodium falciparum*. The mortality rate for transfusion-transmitted malaria is 10%. Exclusion of high-risk donors is the most effective preventive measure currently available.

Transfusion transmission of *T. cruzi*, the cause of Chagas disease, is a problem in areas of the world where the causative agent is endemic, and it has occurred in the United States. Serologic screening for *T. cruzi* infection may be effective when a high proportion of donors have emigrated from such areas. A serologic test has been licensed for the screening of blood donors in the United States and is now required by the FDA.

Anaplasma phagocytophilum, a tick-borne intracellular gram-negative rickettsial bacterium and the cause of human granulocytic anaplasmosis (HGA), has led to eight known cases of transfusion transmission to date; however, there is currently no FDA-licensed test for screening donors or their blood components for HGA.[78]

Prions and Transfusion-Transmitted Disease

Creutzfeldt-Jakob disease (CJD) is an illness caused by proteinaceous particles known as prions. Variant CJD (vCJD) differs from classical CJD in the absence of affected family members, younger age of onset, more rapid progression, and association with consumption of certain animal products. Experimental models and theoretical considerations suggest that transmission by blood components is probable.[79,80] There have been several reports of probable vCJD transmission by blood transfusion.[80,81] B cells and dendritic cells have been suggested to play a crucial role in the development of spongiform encephalopathy, and that possibility has led to the adoption of leukocyte reduction to minimize the risk of transfusion-transmitted vCJD.[82,83] However, no data exist to support universal leukocyte reduction as an efficacious method of preventing the spread of vCJD by transfused blood. At present, there is no practical donor screening test for the abnormal isoform of the prion protein, although progress in test development is being made.[84] Current strategies for reducing the theoretical risk of prion transmission include deferral of donors with a family history of CJD, exposure to risk factors, or residence or blood transfusion in regions where vCJD is endemic. To date, no pathogen inactivation strategy effectively eliminates prions.

Hemovigilance

In 2006, the US Department of Health and Human Services and private-sector blood collection, transfusion, and tissue and organ transplantation organizations initiated a collaboration to monitor adverse events associated with transfusion and transplantation. The hemovigilance module of the CDC National Healthcare Safety Network, the first system used under this collaboration, began to track adverse events of transfusion in February 2010. Reporting tools and other resources are available on the CDC website.[85] Another resource is the AABB Center for Patient Safety, a patient safety organization that analyzes adverse-event data confidentially to identify and promote best practices.[86]

References

1. Food and Drug Administration. Fatalities reported to FDA following blood collection and transfusion: Annual summary for fiscal year 2015. Silver Spring, MD: CBER Office of Communication, Outreach, and Development. [Available at https://www.fda.gov/downloads/BiologicsBloodVaccines/SafetyAvailability/ReportaProblem/TransfusionDonationFatalities/UCM518148.pdf (accessed July 24, 2017).]
2. Unni N, Peddinghaus M, Tormey CA, Stack G. Record fragmentation due to transfusion at multiple health care facilities: A risk factor for delayed hemolytic transfusion reactions. Transfusion 2014;54:98-103.
3. Davenport RD. Hemolytic transfusion reactions. In: Popovsky MA, ed. Transfusion reactions. 4th ed. Bethesda, MD: AABB Press, 2012:1-51.
4. Petz L, Garratty G. The diagnosis of hemolytic anemia. In: Immune hemolytic anemias. 2nd ed. Philadelphia: Churchill Livingstone, 2004:48-9.
5. Gladwin MT. Role of the red blood cell in nitric oxide homeostasis and hypoxic vasodilation. Adv Exp Med Biol 2006;588:189-205.
6. Davenport RD. Inflammatory cytokines in hemolytic transfusion reactions. In: Davenport RD, Snyder EL, eds. Cytokines in transfusion medicine: A primer. Bethesda, MD: AABB Press, 1997:85-97.
7. Butler J, Parker D, Pillai R, et al. Systemic release of neutrophil elastase and tumour necrosis factor alpha following ABO-incompatible blood transfusion. Br J Haematol 1991;79:525-6.
8. Savage WJ, Hod EA. Noninfectious complications of blood transfusion. In: Fung MK, Eder AF, Spitalnik SL, Westhoff CM, eds. Technical manual. 19th ed. Bethesda, MD: AABB, 2017;22:569-98.

9. Davenport RD, Burdick M, Moore SA, Kunkel SL. Cytokine production in IgG-mediated red cell incompatibility. Transfusion 1993;33:19-24.
10. Pierce RN, Reich LM, Mayer K. Hemolysis following platelet transfusions from ABO-incompatible donors. Transfusion 1985;25:60-2.
11. Kim HC, Park CL, Cowan JH, et al. Massive intravascular hemolysis associated with intravenous immunoglobulin in bone marrow transplant recipients. Am J Pediatr Hematol Oncol 1988;10:69-74.
12. Mair B, Benson K. Evaluation of changes in hemoglobin levels associated with ABO-incompatible plasma in apheresis platelets. Transfusion 1998;38:51-5.
13. Petz LD, Calhoun L, Shulman IA, et al. The sickle cell hemolytic transfusion reaction syndrome. Transfusion 1997;37:382-92.
14. King KE, Shirey RS, Lankiewicz MW, et al. Delayed hemolytic transfusion reactions in sickle cell disease: Simultaneous destruction of recipients' red cells. Transfusion 1997;37:376-81.
15. Telen MJ, Combs M. Management of massive delayed hemolytic transfusion reactions in patients with sickle cell disease (abstract). Transfusion 1999;39(Suppl):443S.
16. Win N, Sinha S, Lee E, Mills W. Treatment with intravenous immunoglobulin and steroids may correct severe anemia in hyperhemolytic transfusion reactions: Case report and literature review. Transfus Med Rev 2010;24:64-7.
17. Chadebech P, Habibi AN, Nzouakou R, et al. Delayed hemolytic transfusion reaction in sickle cell disease patients: Evidence of an emerging syndrome with suicidal red blood cell death. Transfusion 2009;49:1785-92.
18. Johnson ST, Fueger JT, Gottschall JL. One center's experience: The serology and drugs associated with drug-induced hemolytic anemia—a new paradigm. Transfusion 2007; 47:697-702.

19. Greninger A, Hess JR. *Clostridium perfringens* sepsis masquerading as a hemolytic transfusion reaction. Transfusion 2017;57:1112.
20. Perkins HA, Payne R, Ferguson J, Wood M. Nonhemolytic febrile transfusion reactions. Quantitative effects of blood components with emphasis on isoantigenic incompatibility of leukocytes. Vox Sang 1966;11:578-99.
21. Wang RR, Triulzi DJ, Qu L. Effects of prestorage versus poststorage leukoreduction on the rate of febrile nonhemolytic transfusion reactions to platelets. Am J Clin Pathol 2012;138:255-9.
22. Mangano MM, Chambers LA, Kruskall MS. Limited efficacy of leukopoor platelets for prevention of febrile transfusion reactions. Am J Clin Pathol 1991;95:733-8.
23. Geiger TL, Howard SC. Acetaminophen and diphenhydramine premedication for allergic and febrile nonhemolytic transfusion reactions: Good prophylaxis or bad practice? Transfus Med Rev 2007;21:1-12.
24. Savage WJ, Tobian AR, Savage JH, et al. Scratching the surface of allergic transfusion reactions. Transfusion 2013;53:1361-71.
25. Tobian AA, Fuller AK, Uqlik K, et al. The impact of platelet additive solution apheresis platelets on allergic transfusion reactions and corrected count increment. Transfusion 2014;54:1523-9.
26. Savage WJ, Hamilton RG, Tobian AA, et al. Defining risk factors and presentations of allergic reactions to platelet transfusion. J Allergy Clin Immunol 2014;133:1772-5.
27. Kennedy L, Case L, Hurd D, et al. A prospective, randomized, double-blind controlled trial of acetaminophen and diphenhydramine pretransfusion medication versus placebo for the prevention of transfusion reactions. Transfusion 2008;48:2285-91.
28. Vyas GN, Perkins HA, Fudenberg HH. Anaphylactoid transfusion reactions associated with anti-IgA. Lancet 1968;ii:12-15.

29. Westhoff CM, Sipherd BD, Wylie DE, Toalson LD. Severe anaphylactic reaction following transfusion of platelets to a patient with anti-Ch. Transfusion 1992; 32:576-9.
30. Koda Y, Watanabe Y, Soejima M, et al. Simple PCR detection of haptoglobin gene deletion in anhaptoglobinemic patients with antihaptoglobin antibody that causes anaphylactic transfusion reactions. Blood 2000;95:1138-43.
31. Davenport RD, Burnie KL, Barr RM. Transfusion management of patients with IgA deficiency and anti-IgA during liver transplantation. Vox Sang 1992;63:247-50.
32. Parmar N, Pendergrast J, Lieberman L, et al. The association of fever with TACO. Vox Sang 2017;112:70-8.
33. Andrzejewski C, Casey MA, Popovsky MA. How we view and approach transfusion associated circulatory overload. Pathogenesis, diagnosis, management, mitigation and prevention. Transfusion 2013;53:3037-47.
34. Kleinman S, Caulfield T, Chan P, et al. Toward an understanding of transfusion-related lung injury: Statement of a consensus panel. Transfusion 2004;44:1774-89.
35. Silliman CC, Ambrusco DR, Boshkov LK. Transfusion-related acute lung injury (TRALI). Blood 2005;105:2266-73.
36. Popovsky MA, Davenport RD. Transfusion-related acute lung injury: Femme fatale? Transfusion 2001;41:312-15.
37. Silliman CC, Paterson AJ, Dickey WO, et al. The association of biologically active lipids with the development of transfusion-related acute lung injury: A retrospective study. Transfusion 1997;37:719-26.
38. Toy P, Hollis-Perry KM, Jun J, et al. Recipients of blood from a donor with multiple HLA antibodies: A lookback study of transfusion-related acute lung injury. Transfusion 2004;44:1683-8.
39. Kopko PM, Marshall CS, MacKenzie MR, et al. Transfusion-related acute lung injury: Report of a clinical lookback investigation. JAMA 2002;287:1968-71.

40. Caudrillier A, Kessenbrock K, Gilliss BM, et al. Platelets induce neutrophil extracellular traps in transfusion-related acute lung injury. J Clin Invest 2012;122:2661-71.
41. TRALI risk mitigation for plasma and whole blood for allogeneic transfusion. Association bulletin #14-02. Bethesda, MD: AABB, 2014.
42. Shiba M, Tadokoro K, Sawanobori M, et al. Activation of the contact system by filtration of platelet concentrates with a negatively charged white cell-removal filter and measurement of venous blood bradykinin level in patients who received filtered platelets. Transfusion 1997;37:45-62.
43. Hild M, Söderström T, Egberg N, Lundahl J. Kinetics of bradykinin levels during and after leucocyte filtration of platelet concentrates. Vox Sang 1998;75:18-25.
44. Mair B, Leparc GF. Hypotensive reactions associated with platelet transfusions and angiotensin-converting enzyme inhibitors. Vox Sang 1998;74:27-30.
45. de Korte D, Marcelis JH, Soeterboek AM. Determination of the degree of bacterial contamination of whole-blood collections using an automated microbe-detection system. Transfusion 2001;41:815-18.
46. Perez P, Salmi LR, Folléa G, et al. Determinants of transfusion-associated bacterial contamination: Results of the French BACTHEM Case-Control Study. Transfusion 2001;41:862-72.
47. Ooley PW, ed. AABB Standards for blood banks and transfusion services. 30th ed. Bethesda, MD: AABB, 2016.
48. Food and Drug Administration. Draft guidance for industry: Bacterial risk control strategies for blood collection establishments and transfusion services to enhance the safety and availability of platelets for transfusion. (March 2016) Silver Spring, MD: CBER Office of Communications, Outreach, and Development, 2016. [Available at https://www.fda.gov/downloads/BiologicsBloodVaccines/GuidanceComplianceRegulatoryInformation/Guidances/Blood/UCM425952.pdf (accessed July 24, 2017).]

49. Eder A, Kennedy J, Dy B, et al. Bacterial screening of apheresis platelets and the residual risk of septic transfusion reactions: The American Red Cross experience (2004-2006). Transfusion 2007;47:1134-42.
50. Dzik WH, Kirkley SA. Citrate toxicity during massive blood transfusion. Transfus Med Rev 1988;2:76-94.
51. Driscoll DF, Bistrian BR, Jenkins RL, et al. Development of metabolic alkalosis after massive transfusion during orthotopic liver transplantation. Crit Care Med 1987;15: 905-8.
52. Zimring JC. Principles of red blood cell alloimmunization and autoantibody formation and function. In: Hillyer CD, Silberstein L, Ness PM, et al, eds. Blood banking and transfusion medicine: Basic principles and practice. 2nd ed. Philadelphia: Churchill Livingstone, 2007:43-52.
53. Kohan AI, Niborski RC, Rey JA, et al. High-dose intravenous immunoglobulin in non-ABO transfusion incompatibility. Vox Sang 1994;67:195-8.
54. Mueller-Eckhardt C. Post-transfusion purpura. Br J Haematol 1986;64:419-24.
55. Laursen B, Morling N, Rosenkvist J, et al. Post-transfusion purpura treated with plasma exchange by Haemonetics cell separator. Acta Med Scand 1978;203:539-43.
56. Linden JV, Pisciotto PT. Transfusion-associated graft-versus-host disease and blood irradiation. Transfus Med Rev 1992;6:116-23.
57. Holland PV. Prevention of transfusion-associated graft-vs-host disease. Arch Pathol Lab Med 1989;113:285-91.
58. Thaler M, Shamiss A, Orgad S, et al. The role of blood from HLA homozygous donors in fatal transfusion-associated graft-versus-host disease after open heart surgery. N Engl J Med 1989;321:25-8.
59. Shivdasani RA, Haluska FG, Dock NL, et al. Graft-versus-host disease associated with transfusion of blood from unrelated HLA-homozygous donors. N Engl J Med 1993; 328:766-70.

60. Krenger W, Ferrara JLM. Dysregulation of cytokines during graft-versus-host disease. J Hematother 1996;5:3-14.
61. Moroff G, Luban NLC. The irradiation of blood and blood components to prevent graft-versus-host disease: Technical issues and guidelines. Transfus Med Rev 1997;11:15-26.
62. Hoffbrand AV, Cohen A, Hershko C. Role of deferiprone in chelation therapy for transfusional iron overload. Blood 2003;102:17-24.
63. Marcus CS, Huehns ER. Transfusional iron overload. Clin Lab Haematol 1985;7:195-212.
64. Delea T, Edelsberg J, Sofrygin O, et al. Consequences and costs of noncompliance with iron chelation treatment in patients with transfusion dependent thalassemia: A literature review. Transfusion 2007;47:1919-29.
65. Linden J, Kaplan H, Murphy MT. Fatal air embolism due to perioperative blood recovery. Anesth Analg 1997;84:422-6.
66. Stramer SL, Galel SA. Infectious disease screening. In: Fung MK, Eder AF, Spitalnik SL, Westhoff CM, eds. Technical manual. 19th ed. Bethesda, MD: AABB, 2017;7:161-206.
67. Stramer S, Wend U, Candotti D, et al. Nucleic acid testing to detect HBV infection in blood donors. N Engl J Med 2011;364:236-47.
68. Nelson KE. Transmission of hepatitis E virus by transfusion: What is the risk? Transfusion 2014;54:8-10.
69. Iwamoto M, Jernigan DB, Guasch A, et al. Transmission of West Nile virus from an organ donor to four transplant recipients. N Engl J Med 2003;348:2196-203.
70. Pealer LN, Marfin AA, Lanciotti RS, et al. Transmission of West Nile virus through blood transfusion in the United States, 2002. N Engl J Med 2003;349:1236-45.
71. Song BH, Yun SI, Woolley M, Lee YM. Zika virus: History, epidemiology, transmission, and clinical presentation. J Neuroimmunol 2017;308:50-64.

72. Motta IJF, Spencer BR, Cordeiro da Silva SG, et al. Evidence for transmission of Zika virus by platelet transfusion. N Engl J Med 2016;375:1101-3.
73. Larsson S, Söderberg-Nauclér C, Wang FZ, Möller E. Cytomegalovirus DNA can be detected in peripheral blood mononuclear cells from all seropositive and most seronegative healthy blood donors over time. Transfusion 1998;38: 271-8.
74. Bowden RA, Slichter SJ, Sayers M, et al. A comparison of filtered leukocyte-reduced and cytomegalovirus (CMV)-seronegative blood products for the prevention of transfusion-associated CMV infection after marrow transplantation. Blood 1995;86:3598-603.
75. Koenigbauer UF, Eastland T, Day JW. Clinical illness due to parvovirus B19 infection after infusion of solvent/detergent-treated pooled plasma. Transfusion 2000;40:1203-6.
76. Cushing M, Shaz B. Transfusion-transmitted babesiosis: Achieving successful mitigation while balancing cost and donor loss. Transfusion 2012;52:1404-07.
77. Mungai M, Tegtmeier G, Chamberland M, Parise M. Transfusion-transmitted malaria in the United States from 1963 through 1999. N Engl J Med 2001;344:1973-8.
78. Fine AB, Sweeney JD, Nixon CP, Knoll BM. Transfusion-transmitted anaplasmosis from a leukoreduced platelet pool. Transfusion 2016;56:699-704.
79. Houston F, Foster JD, Chong A, et al. Transmission of BSE by blood transfusion in sheep. Lancet 2000;356:999-1000.
80. Llewelyn CA, Hewitt PE, Knight RSG, et al. Possible transmission of variant Creutzfeldt-Jakob disease by blood transfusion. Lancet 2004;363:417-21.
81. Peden AH, Head MW, Ritchie DL, et al. Preclinical vCJD after blood transfusion in a PRNP codon 129 heterozygous patient. Lancet 2004;364:527-9.
82. Klein MA, Frigg R, Flechsig E, et al. A crucial role for B cells in neuroinvasive scrapie. Nature 1997;390:687-90.

83. Klein MA, Frigg R, Raeber AJ, et al. PrP expression in B lymphocytes is not required for prion neuroinvasion. Nat Med 1998;4:1429-33.
84. MacGregor I. Prion protein and developments in its detection. Transfus Med 2001;11:3-14.
85. Centers for Disease Control and Prevention. National Healthcare Safety Network (NHSN): Blood safety surveillance. Atlanta, GA: CDC, 2016. [Available at https://www.cdc.gov/nhsn/acute-care-hospital/bio-hemo/ (accessed July 24, 2017).]
86. AABB hemovigilance. Bethesda, MD: AABB, 2017. [Available at http://www.aabb.org/research/hemovigilance/Pages/default.aspx (accessed July 24, 2017).]

THERAPEUTIC APHERESIS

Description

Therapeutic apheresis involves the separation of a patient's whole blood to remove and, in many cases, to replace a portion of the blood that contains an abnormal constituent, to achieve a clinical benefit.[1] Apheresis procedures are defined by the blood component removed and/or exchanged: cytapheresis is directed toward any cellular element and includes leukocytapheresis, lymphocytapheresis, erythrocytapheresis, and plateletpheresis, whereas therapeutic plasma exchange (TPE) targets plasma. Although partial blood exchanges can be performed manually by using phlebotomy and simple transfusion, the use of automated cell-separation instruments permits the processing of larger quantities of blood safely, efficiently, and in a more targeted manner.[2]

The American Society for Apheresis (ASFA) categorizes the utility of therapeutic apheresis using published evidence with respect to various diseases in the "Guidelines on the Use of Therapeutic Apheresis in Clinical Practice—Evidence-Based Approach from the Writing Committee of the American Society for Apheresis."[3] This document provides the summation of clinical studies and offers a useful resource for practicing clinicians and apheresis providers when they are contemplating using apheresis as a therapeutic modality. The ASFA categories, which are used to rank the clinical utility of apheresis, are outlined in Table 16. In addition to ASFA categorization, the GRADE system (Grading of Recommendations Assessment, Development, and

Table 16. American Society for Apheresis Indication Categories[3]

Category	Description
I	Disorders for which apheresis is accepted as first-line therapy, either as a primary stand-alone treatment or in conjunction with other modes of treatment.
II	Disorders for which apheresis is accepted as second-line therapy, either as a stand-alone treatment or in conjunction with other modes of treatment.
III	Optimum role of apheresis therapy is not established. Decision making should be individualized.
IV	Disorders in which published evidence demonstrates or suggests apheresis to be ineffective or harmful. IRB approval is desirable if apheresis treatment is undertaken in these circumstances.

IRB = institutional review board.

Evaluation) is also applied to each disease state to indicate the level of evidence that is available.[4] Table 17 categorizes some of the diseases most commonly treated by therapeutic apheresis.

Indications

Cytapheresis

Therapeutic cytapheresis can be used to reduce excessive or abnormal cellular elements in the blood. This technique is typically employed in emergency situations when there is imminent

Table 17. Common Diagnoses for Which Therapeutic Apheresis Is Performed*

Disease Name	ASFA Category
Acute disseminated encephalomyelitis, steroid refractory	II
Acute inflammatory demyelinating polyradiculoneuropathy (Guillain-Barré syndrome)	I
• After intravenous immune globulin	III
Acute liver failure	
• High-volume plasma exchange	I
• Plasma exchange	III
ANCA rapidly progressing glomerulonephritis (Wegener), dialysis independence	III
• Diffuse alveolar hemorrhage (DAH)†	I
• Dialysis dependence	I
Antiglomerular basement membrane disease (Goodpasture syndrome)	I
• Dialysis independence	I
• DAH†	I
• Dialysis dependence and no DAH	III
Catastrophic antiphospholipid syndrome†	II
Chronic inflammatory demyelinating polyradiculoneuropathy (CIDP)	I
Familial hypercholesterolemia, homozygous	
• Homozygous	I
• Heterozygous	II
Focal segmental glomerulosclerosis	
• Recurrent in transplanted kidney	I
• Steroid-resistant native kidney	III
Hyperleukocytosis, leukostasis†	II
• Prophylactic or secondary	III

(Continued)

Table 17. Common Diagnoses for Which Therapeutic Apheresis Is Performed* (Continued)

Disease Name	ASFA Category
• Sympthomatic	II
Hyperviscosity in monoclonal gammopathies, symptomatic or prophylactic for rituximab	I
Lipoprotein (a) hyperlipoproteinemia	II
Liver transplantation	
• Desensitization, ABO incompatible, living donor	I
• Desensitization, ABO incompatible, deceased donor	III
Lung transplantation	
• Bronchiolitis obliterans syndrome (ECP)	II
• Antibody-mediated rejection and desensitization	III
Multiple sclerosis	
• Acute central nervous system inflammatory demyelinating disease (TPE; immunoadsorption)	II, III
• Chronic progressive	III
Myasthenia gravis, moderate-to-severe or before thymectomy	I
Myeloma cast nephropathy	II
Neuromyelitis optica (Devic syndrome)	
• Acute	II
• Maintenance	III
Paraproteinemic demyelinating polyneuropathies	
• IgG, IgA, IgM (TPE)	I
• Multiple myeloma	III
Polycythemia vera	I
• Secondary erythrocytosis	III
Renal transplantation, ABO compatible	
• Antibody-mediated rejection	I

Table 17. Common Diagnoses for Which Therapeutic Apheresis Is Performed* (Continued)

Disease Name	ASFA Category
• Desensitization, living donor	I
• Desensitization, deceased donor	III
Renal transplantation, ABO incompatible	
• Desensitization, living donor	I
• Antibody-mediated rejection (TPE, IA)	II
Sepsis with multiorgan failure	III
Sickle cell disease	
• Acute stroke†	I
• Severe acute chest syndrome†	II
• Acute priapism, multiorgan failure, splenic or hepatic sequestration†	III
• Nonacute, recurrent stroke prevention	III
• Nonacute, veno-occlusive pain crisis	I
• Preoperative management	III
Thrombocytosis, symptomatic	II
Thrombotic microangiopathy, complement mediated	
• Atypical HUS (complement gene mutations)	III
• Factor H autoantibodies	I
Thrombotic microangiopathy, Shiga-toxin mediated (HUS)	
• Severe neurological symptoms	III
• Streptococcus	III
Thrombotic thrombocytopenic purpura†	I
Voltage-gated potassium channel antibodies	II

*Adapted from Schwartz et al.[3] The table does not reflect every diagnosis that has been categorized.
†The diagnosis may be a potential apheresis emergency.
ASFA = American Society for Apheresis; ANCA = antineutrophil cytoplasmic antibody; ECP = extracorporeal photopheresis; TPE = therapeutic plasma exchange; HUS = hemolytic uremic syndrome.

or ongoing end-organ damage resulting from the cell burden and conventional therapies are ineffective or too slow to take effect. The resulting postprocedure change in cell counts is temporary and may, or may not, affect long-term clinical outcome.

Erythrocytapheresis or red cell exchange by apheresis has been used to manage acute or severe complications of sickle cell disease, such as stroke and acute chest syndrome, by reducing the level of hemoglobin S to less than 30%.[5] For long-term prevention (secondary prophylaxis) of stroke or silent cerebral infarct, reducing the level of hemoglobin S to less than 30% to 50% with a chronic schedule of apheresis has been successful.[6,7] The use of erythrocytapheresis is effective in managing and preventing iron overload associated with chronic transfusion in patients with sickle cell disease.[8] Erythrocytapheresis is less commonly used for other indications; it has been used to treat overwhelming parasitic infections (malaria and babesiosis). Evidence suggests that red cell exchange is effective as a second-line therapy to treat severe malaria with red cell parasitemia >10%.[9,10] It has been used in the setting of immune-mediated hemolysis, hemochromatosis, and polycythemia vera/erythrocytosis when rapid hematocrit normalization is needed.[11,12]

Leukocytapheresis may be useful in the management of hyperleukocytosis with leukostasis. Symptomatic leukostasis usually affects the central nervous system and/or pulmonary system when myeloblasts exceed 70,000 to 100,000/μL; the procedure causes cytoreduction by 30% to 60% while definitive therapy is being initiated. The cell subtype, and thus cellular deformability, is important. The efficacy of leukocytapheresis for leukostasis is supported by some, but not all, retrospective studies, which suggest early death is prevented, but overall survival is not affected, in adult acute myelogenous leukemia.[13] Children with acute lymphoblastic leukemia do not usually have symptoms of leukostasis if the leukocyte count is <400,000/μL, and apheresis does not offer benefit over aggressive chemotherapy.[14] Patients with acute promyelocytic leukemia do not appear to benefit.

In patients with myeloproliferative disorders and severe symptomatic thrombocytosis, plateletpheresis can be useful in the prevention of thrombotic and hemorrhagic complications by acutely lowering the platelet count. An improvement in bleeding may be abrogation of acquired von Willebrand disease seen when platelet counts are >1,500,000/μL, because platelets at this level promote von Willebrand factor clearance.[15] Generally, plateletpheresis is used when the platelet count exceeds 1,000,000/μL or with clinical signs of microvascular ischemia. Typically, the platelet count is transiently lowered by 30% to 60% after a single procedure.[16-18] Plateletpheresis is uncommonly required because of the effectiveness of therapeutic agents such as anagrelide, hydroxyurea, and interferon alpha.[3]

Therapeutic Plasma Exchange

Plasmapheresis refers to the separation of plasma by apheresis, such as for plasma donation, and does not include replacement. Plasma exchange includes the removal of the plasma and replacement of it by using a fluid such as albumin, saline, human plasma, or a mixture of fluids. The goal of the therapy is to remove antibodies or toxic mediators and/or to replace the plasma component of the blood. TPE has found widespread clinical application in the management of a variety of autoimmune, hematologic, renal, metabolic, and neurologic disorders. Most TPE regimens include the processing of 1.0 to 1.5 plasma volumes for each of five to six procedures performed over a 10- to 14-day period. The volume exchanged and the number and frequency of procedures are dependent on the disease indication.[3] The removal of large amounts of plasma necessitates concurrent replacement with colloid, crystalloid, or a combination of solutions. Albumin (5%) is the most commonly used replacement solution. Plasma may also be used. In patients experiencing active hemorrhage or with a high risk of bleeding, such as an imminent or recent invasive procedure, plasma may be used as part of the replacement fluid solution to avoid transient dilutional coagulopathy resulting from the use of albumin or colloid replacement alone.

TPE is commonly used in neurologic diseases, usually to target immunologic disorders, together with other immunomodulatory therapies. Myasthenia gravis and severe acute inflammatory demyelinating polyradiculoneuropathy are two of the more common diagnoses treated with TPE.[19] Neuromyelitis optica (NMO) is an inflammatory demyelinating disease caused by an autoantibody to the aquaporin-4 receptor.[20] Since the discovery of the etiologic cause of NMO, other encephalopathies and paraproteinemic neurologic syndromes have been found to be caused by specific receptor antibodies such as those to voltage-gated potassium channels or synaptic proteins, which may be effectively treated with TPE.[21]

There are numerous hematologic conditions treated with TPE.[3] Patients with thrombotic thrombocytopenic purpura (TTP) are treated with daily TPE using plasma as replacement until there is normalization of the platelet count and lactate dehydrogenase.[22] For most of the other presentations of thrombotic microangiopathy (TMA), such as atypical hemolytic uremic syndrome (aHUS, also called complement-mediated HUS) and drug-induced TMA, other therapeutic treatments are favored as first-line therapy. However, TPE may be effective in certain settings.[22-27]

Plasma exchange is used in conjunction with immunosuppression regimens for removal of HLA and ABO antibodies in the setting of hematopoietic stem cell transplantation and solid organ transplantation, typically kidney, liver, and heart. The procedure can be used before transplantation to decrease the chance of hyperacute rejection, or after the transplantation when there is humoral rejection.

Selective Lipid Removal (Lipid Apheresis)

Selective adsorption columns combined with apheresis technology have been used to remove targeted substances. Lipid apheresis can be used to reduce apolipoprotein-B-containing lipoproteins, including low-density lipoprotein (LDL) and lipoprotein (a), with conservation of high-density lipoprotein.[28] Lipid apheresis consists of plasma separation followed by one of the following: adsorption of LDL onto negatively charged dextran-sulfate-coated or LDL-antibody-coated sepharose beads, precipitation of LDL by negatively charged heparin, or removal of LDL by filtration. Procedures are usually performed every 2 weeks, and a single procedure can transiently lower the LDL cholesterol by 70% to 80%. LDL apheresis is approved to treat steroid-refractory focal and segmental glomerulosclerosis in children. It has also been used to treat the lipid damage to the kidney in focal and segmental glomerulonephritis.

Extracorporeal Photopheresis

Extracorporeal photopheresis (ECP), or photopheresis, has been found to be efficacious in selected malignant and autoimmune disorders. The technique involves collecting blood leukocytes via apheresis technology and then exposing the cells to the drug 8-methoxypsoralen, which binds to DNA inside the cells and, upon stimulation with ultraviolet light (UVA), prevents DNA replication and RNA transcription. This inhibits lymphocyte proliferation and induces apoptosis of the treated cells after reinfusion back to the patient.[29] ECP has become standard therapy for advanced erythrodermic forms of cutaneous T-cell lymphoma and Sézary syndrome. It is also commonly used for steroid-resistant chronic graft-vs-host disease following allogeneic hematopoietic stem cell transplantation.[30] ECP has shown promise in the management of solid organ transplant rejection and the prevention and management of acute graft-vs-host disease.[3]

Procedural Considerations

Vascular access is an important clinical issue for patients that require apheresis.[31] Whenever possible, antecubital peripheral venous access should be used because of its lower risk. Peripheral venous access must be able to accommodate the flow rate (≥ 1 mL/kg/minute) required during the apheresis procedure. In addition, the patient's arms must be relatively immobilized for several hours to ensure continuation of apheresis and to lower the risk of venous penetration and nerve injury. Young age, altered mental status, inability to cooperate, frequent need to urinate, decreased muscle tone, and hyperviscosity may preclude the use of peripheral venous access. If a central line is required, specialized noncollapsible types (eg, dialysis catheters) must be used. Internal jugular and subclavian veins are common choices for central access. Fistulas, grafts, and specialized ports are also used for vascular access; these types of central access require surgical or interventional radiology placement. In emergent apheresis, a femoral central venous catheter poses no risk of pneumothorax and, if bleeding should occur, pressure on the entry point can be used and may be preferable in a thrombocytopenic patient.[32] The femoral location has a higher risk of infection and thrombosis. Tunneled central access catheters have lower rates of infection and are preferred for longer intervals of therapy. Saline, heparin, acid-citrate-dextrose A (ACD-A), or sometimes tissue plasminogen activator must be used to maintain catheter patency.

Priming of the apheresis circuit with red cells may be necessary for patients weighing less than 25 kg or patients with severe anemia, because of the extracorporeal shift of red cells in the apheresis circuit, which effectively decreases the patient's intraprocedure hematocrit and, thus, oxygen-carrying capacity.

Complications of Therapeutic Apheresis

Complications of apheresis can be related to the procedure, replacement fluid, or intravenous access. Complications related to an apheresis procedure can occur during and after apheresis. The reported incidence of adverse events or complications ranges from 4.75% to 55% in different series, suggesting differences in how adverse events were collected and graded.[33,34]

Intravenous-access-related complications can be seen with both peripheral and central access routes. Hematoma and nerve injury can occur after venipuncture. Risks associated with central catheters include bleeding, infection, catheter thrombosis, air embolism, pulmonary embolism, cardiac arrhythmias, and cardiorespiratory arrest. In patients receiving apheresis in outpatient clinics, catheter care must be taught or assigned to home health care providers to ensure the line remains usable and does not become infected.

Citrate, found in the ACD solution that is commonly used as anticoagulant in the apheresis circuit, chelates ionized calcium temporarily to prevent coagulation factor activation in the apheresis device. One of the most common complications during apheresis is citrate-related hypocalcemia, which manifests frequently as perioral tingling, numbness, paresthesias, or muscle cramping. Rarely, severe hypocalcemia may be associated with cardiac dysrhythmias. Hypocalcemia is more likely in large-volume procedures or when plasma is used as the replacement solution. Symptoms can be managed or prevented (prophylaxis) with calcium replacement (intravenous or oral calcium). Citrate- related toxicity is often transient, because the liver and kidneys can metabolize citrate quickly, and it usually resolves within minutes to hours of the cessation of apheresis. Persons with liver failure may be especially susceptible to citrate toxicity, as are patients who are unable to report early symptoms. Monitoring of ionized calcium may be medically prudent in these cases, such as in pediatric patients.

Flushing and hypotension have been reported in patients taking angiotensin-converting enzyme (ACE) inhibitors who receive albumin replacement during standard apheresis.[35] ACE inhibitors block the degradation of bradykinins that are present in albumin solutions. Rare reactions include seizures, anaphylaxis (with plasma infusions), and cardiorespiratory arrest.

Hypotension is the most common side effect in patients undergoing lipid apheresis. Patients should discontinue taking ACE inhibitors before a procedure. Holding other antihypertensive medications before an apheresis procedure should be evaluated on a case-by-case basis.

Fluid shifts occurring during apheresis can lead to hypotension, volume depletion, volume overload, or vasovagal reactions. Depending on the symptom, the fluid balance and amount exchanged may need to be altered to maintain blood pressure. Depletion of coagulation factors may increase the risk for bleeding and, rarely, thrombosis. Dilutional coagulopathy can be mitigated by using partial plasma replacement at the end of the procedure. Complications related to apheresis replacement fluids include allergic reactions, transfusion reactions, and transfusion-transmitted diseases if patients receive blood components. Rarely, allergic-type reactions can occur from the ethylene oxide coating of the sterile tubing.

Because of the higher risk of infection with progressive depletion of immunoglobulins after undergoing many serial TPE procedures, some patients may benefit from intravenous immune globulin infusion when immunoglobulin G (IgG) levels are reduced below 200 mg/dL. Chronic erythrocytapheresis procedures can be used to reduce iron overload, but can also lead to iron-deficiency anemia.

Concentrations of some drugs, particularly those that are protein bound (eg, antibiotics, anticoagulants, and sedatives), and immune globulin preparations may be lowered by TPE. Whenever possible, daily medications should be administered *after* TPE. To avoid erroneous laboratory results caused by hemodilution or passively acquired antibodies from donor plasma, diagnostic and/or serologic tests should be performed on blood samples *before* apheresis. This is particularly important when testing for ADAMTS13 in a patient with suspected TTP.

References

1. Weinstein R. Basic principles of therapeutic blood exchange. In: McLeod BC, Szczepiorkowski ZM, Weinstein R, Winters JL, eds. Apheresis: Principles and practice. 3rd ed. Bethesda, MD: AABB Press, 2010:269-94.
2. Brecher M. Therapeutic apheresis: Why we do what we do. J Clin Apher 2002;17:207-11.
3. Schwartz J, Padmanabhan A, Aqui N, et al. Guidelines on the use of therapeutic apheresis in clinical practice—evidence-based approach from the Writing Committee of the American Society for Apheresis: The seventh special issue. J Clin Apher 2016;31:149-338.
4. Guyatt G, Gutterman D, Baumann MH, et al. Grading strength of recommendations and quality of evidence in clinical guidelines: Report from an American College of Chest Physicians task force. Chest 2006;129:174-81.
5. US Department of Health and Human Services, National Institutes of Health. Evidence-based management of sickle cell disease. Expert panel report, 2014. Bethesda, MD: National Heart, Lung, and Blood Institute, 2014.
6. Singer ST, Quirolo K, Nishi K, et al. Erythrocytapheresis for chronically transfused children with sickle cell disease: An effective method for maintaining a low hemoglobin S level and reducing iron overload. J Clin Apher 1999;14:122-5.
7. DeBaun MR, Gordon M, McKinstry RC, et al. Controlled trial of transfusions for silent cerebral infarcts in sickle cell anemia. N Engl J Med 2014;371:699-710.
8. Kim HC, Dugan NP, Silber JH, et al. Erythrocytapheresis therapy to reduce iron overload in chronically transfused patients with sickle cell disease. Blood 1994;83:1136-42.
9. Tan KR, Wiegand RE, Auguin PM. Exchange transfusion for severe malaria: Evidence base and literature review. Clin Infect Dis 2013;57:923-8.

10. Shaz BH, Schwartz J, Winters JL, et al. ASFA guidelines support use of red cell exchange for severe malaria with high parasitemia. Clin Infect Dis 2014;58:302-3.
11. Balint B, Ostojic G, Pavlovic M, et al. Cytapheresis in the treatment of cell-affected blood disorders and abnormalities. Transfus Apher Sci 2006;35:25-31.
12. Rusak T, Ciborowski M, Uchimiak-Owieczko A, et al. Evaluation of hemostatic balance in blood from patients with polycythemia vera by means of thromboelastography: The effect of isovolemic erythrocytapheresis. Platelets 2012;23:455-62.
13. Ganzel C, Becker J, Mintz PD, et al. Hyperleukocytosis, leukostasis and leukapheresis: Practice management. Blood Rev 2012;26:117-22.
14. Nguyen R, Jeha S, Zhou Y, et al. The role of leukapheresis in the current management of hyperleukocytosis in newly diagnosed childhood acute lymphoblastic leukemia. Pediatr Blood Cancer 2016;63:1546-51.
15. van Genderen PJ, Prins FJ, Lucas IS, et al. Decreased half-life time of plasma von Willebrand factor collagen binding activity in essential thrombocythaemia: Normalization after cytoreduction of the increased platelet count. Br J Haematol 1997;99:832-6.
16. Greist A. The role of blood component removal in essential and reactive thrombocytosis. Ther Apher 2002;6:36-44.
17. Grima KM. Therapeutic apheresis in hematological and oncological diseases. J Clin Apher 2000;15:28-52.
18. Adami R. Therapeutic thrombocytapheresis: A review of 132 patients. Int J Artif Organs 1993;16(Suppl 5):183-4.
19. Cortese I, Chaudry V, So YT, et al. Evidence-based guideline update: Plasmapheresis in neurologic disorders. Report of the Therapeutics and Technology Assessment Subcommittee of the American Academy of Neurology. Neurology 2011;76:294-300.
20. Watanabe S, Nakashima I, Misu T, et al. Therapeutic efficacy of plasma exchange in NMO-IgG-positive patients with neuromyelitis optica. Mult Scler 2007;13:128-32.

21. Jaben EA, Winters JL. Plasma exchange as a therapeutic option in patients with neurologic symptoms due to antibodies to voltage-gated potassium channels: A report of five cases and review of the literature. J Clin Apher 2012; 27:267-73.
22. Scully M, Hunt BJ, Benjamin S, et al. Guidelines on the diagnosis and management of thrombotic thrombocytopenic purpura and other thrombotic microangiopathies. Br J Haematol 2012;158:323-35.
23. Menne J, Nitschke M, Stingele R, et al. Validation of treatment strategies for enterohaemorrhagic *Escherichia coli* O104:H4 induced haemolytic uraemic syndrome: Case-control study. Br Med J 2012;345:e4565.
24. Zuber J, Fakhouri F, Roumenina LT, et al. Use of eculizumab for atypical hemolytic uraemic syndrome and C3 glomerulopathies. Nat Rev Nephrol 2012;8:643-57.
25. Kreuter J, Winters JL. Drug-associated thrombotic micro angiopathies. Semin Thromb Hemost 2012;38:839-44.
26. Kennedy GA, Kearey N, Bleakley S, et al. Transplantation-associated thrombotic microangiopathy: Effect of concomitant GVHD on efficacy of therapeutic plasma exchange. Bone Marrow Transplant 2010;45:699-704.
27. Greinacher A, Friesecke S, Abel P, et al. Treatment of severe neurological deficits with IgG depletion through immunoadsorption in patients with *Escherichia coli* O104:H4-associated haemolytic uraemic syndrome: A prospective trial. Lancet 2011;378:1166-73.
28. Kroon AA, van Asten WN, Stalenhoef AF. Effect of apheresis of low-density lipoprotein on peripheral vascular disease in hypercholesterolemic patients with coronary artery disease. Ann Intern Med 1996;125:945-54.
29. Edelson RL. Transimmunization: The science catches up to the clinical success. Transfus Apher Sci 2002;26:177-80.
30. Flowers ME, Apperley JF, van Besien K, et al. A multicenter prospective phase 2 randomized study of extracor-

poreal photopheresis for treatment of chronic graft-versus-host disease. Blood 2008;112:2667-74.
31. Kalantari K. The choice of vascular access for therapeutic apheresis. J Clin Apher 2012;27:153-9.
32. Cooling L, Hoffmann S, Webb D, et al. Procedure-related complications and adverse events associated with pediatric autologous peripheral blood stem cell collection. J Clin Apher 2017;32:35-48.
33. McLeod BC, Sniecinski I, Ciavarella D, et al. Frequency of immediate adverse effects associated with therapeutic apheresis. Transfusion 1999;39:282-8.
34. Michon B, Moghrabi A, Winikoff R, et al. Complications of apheresis in children. Transfusion 2007;47:1837-42.
35. Owen HG, Brecher ME. Atypical reactions associated with use of angiotensin-converting enzyme inhibitors and apheresis. Transfusion 1994;34:891-4.

INDEX

Page numbers in italics refer to figures and tables.

A

ABC (Assessment of Blood Consumption) score, 202, *205*
Abciximab (ReoPro), acquired platelet disorder due to, 117
ABO compatibility, 142, *144*
  in massive transfusion, 206-207
  in solid organ transplantation, 149
ABO incompatibility
  acute hemolytic transfusion reaction due to, 222
  in massive transfusion, 204-206
  of platelet components, 15, 17
  in solid organ transplantation, 149
ABO type, screen, and crossmatch, 142-144, *143, 144*
ABO-mismatched allogeneic hematopoietic progenitor cell transplantation, 146, *147-148*
ACE (angiotensin-converting enzyme) inhibitors with therapeutic apheresis, 267-268
Activated clotting time (ACT), intraoperative monitoring of, 183
Activated partial thromboplastin time (aPTT), 86-87
Activated prothrombin complex concentrates (aPCCs, FEIBA), *56*, 65, 103

Acute hemolytic transfusion reactions (AHTRs), 221-225
  clinical presentation of, 223-225
  diagnosis of, 222-223
  drug-induced, 230
  etiology and pathogenesis of, 222-223
  extravascular, 223-225, *226*
  intravascular, 222, *224, 226*
  nonimmune, 231
  severity of, 223
  sickle cell, 225-230
  workup for, 223-225, *224-225*
Acute normovolemic hemodilution (ANH), 179
Acute transfusion reactions, 221-238, *226-229*
  allergic, *227*, 232-233
  due to bacterial contamination, *224-225, 229*, 236-237
  defined, 221
  drug-induced hemolysis as, 230
  extravascular hemolytic, 223-225, *226*
  febrile nonhemolytic, *227*, 231-232
  hemolytic, 221-225
  hypotension as, *229*, 235-236
  immune, *224, 226*
  intravascular hemolytic, 222, *224, 226*
  metabolic, 238

273

nonimmune hemolysis as, 231
sickle cell hemolytic, 225-230
due to thermal effects, 237-238
transfusion-associated circulatory overload (TACO) as, *228,* 233-234
transfusion-related acute lung injury (TRALI) as, *228,* 234-235
workup of, *224-225*
ADAMTS13 deficiency, 128
Additive solution (AS)
platelet, *3,* 12-13
red cells, *2,* 10, 11
whole blood, 5
Adverse effects. *See* Transfusion reactions
Adynovate (recombinant Factor VIII PEGylated), 59
Afstyla (recombinant Factor VIII single chain), 59
Aggrastat (tirofiban), acquired platelet disorder due to, 117
AHF. *See* Antihemophilic factor (AHF)
AHTRs. *See* Acute hemolytic transfusion reactions (AHTRs)
Air embolism, 242
Albumin, *57,* 67-68
Allergic transfusion reactions, *227,* 232-233
Alpha$_2$-plasmin inhibitor deficiency, 109-110
Alphanate (von Willebrand factor-containing Factor VIII concentrate), 59, 95-97, *97, 100*
Alprolix (Factor IX concentrates), *54,* 61-62, 102
Amotosalen/UVA light phototherapy system, 36-37, 38
Anaphylactic transfusion reactions, *227,* 232-233
Anaplasmosis, human granulocytic, 246
Anemia
defined, 172
evaluating preoperative, 172-173
in premature infants, 155
Angiomax (bivalirudin), 113
Angiotensin-converting enzyme (ACE) inhibitors with therapeutic apheresis, 267-268
ANH (acute normovolemic hemodilution), 179
Antibody screening in obstetric patients, 151
Anticoagulant(s), 113-114
Anticoagulant systems, natural, in hemostasis, 84
Antifibrinolytic drugs, 98, 121-122
Antihemophilic factor (AHF), *4,* 24-26, 58
for fibrinogen deficiency, 109
for hemophilia A (Factor VIII deficiency), 98-99
for von Willebrand disease, 96
Antiphospholipid syndrome, 125-126
Antiplatelet agents, acquired platelet disorder due to, 116-117

Antithrombin (AT)
    in hemostasis, 84
    concentrate (Atryn), *56,* 63-64
    deficiency, 124-125
aPCCs (activated prothrombin complex concentrates), *56,* 65, 103
Apheresis, therapeutic. *See* Therapeutic apheresis
Apheresis platelets, *3,* 12, 16, 27
Apheresis technology, 1-5
Apixaban (Eliquis), 114
aPTT (activated partial thromboplastin time), 86-87
Argatroban, 113
Arixtra (fondaparinux), 112
ASPEN syndrome, 159
Aspirin, 90-91, 116
Assessment of Blood Consumption (ABC) score, 202, *205*
AT. *See* Antithrombin
Atryn (antithrombin concentrate), *56,* 63-64
Autologous blood donation, preoperative, 176-177

B

Babesia, 242, 246
Bacterial contamination, acute transfusion reactions due to, *224-225, 229,* 236-237
Bebulin VH. *See* Prothrombin complex concentrates (PCCs, Bebulin VH, Profilnine SD, Kcentra)
Berinert (C1 esterase inhibitors), 66-67
Bivalirudin (Angiomax), 113

Bleeding disorders. *See* Hemostatic disorders
Blood administration, 161-165
    blood component identification for, 161-162
    blood warming for, 163
    with concomitant use of intravenous solutions, 164
    filters in, 165
    infusion devices in, 163-164
    time limits for, 162
Blood collection system, 1-5
Blood component(s), 1-38
    commonly used, *2-4*
    cryoprecipitated antihemophilic factor as, *4,* 24-26
    granulocytes as, *4,* 17-20
    identification of, 162
    modification of, 26-35
        freezing and deglycerolization as, *3,* 34-35
        irradiation as, 30-33, *32*
        leukocyte reduction as, *2, 3,* 26-30
        washing as, *2,* 33-34
    and oxygen therapeutics, 35-36
    pathogen inactivation in, 36-38
    plasma, *4,* 20-24
    platelet, *3,* 12-17
    red cell, *2,* 9-11
    time limits for infusing, 162
    whole blood as, 5-9, *6-7*
Blood component resuscitation in trauma and massive bleeding. *See* Massive transfusion (MT)

Blood component therapy, concept of, 1-5
Blood component transfusion strategies in massive hemorrhage, 200-202
Blood donation, preoperative autologous, 176-177
Blood filters, 165
Blood loss, prevention of excessive iatrogenic, 184
Blood order schedule, surgical, 177-179
Blood pumps, 163-164
Blood recovery
 intraoperative, 179-180
 postoperative, 184-185
Blood typing, 141-144, *143, 144*
Blood utilization review, 186-187
Blood vessels in hemostasis, 81-82
Blood warming, 163

C

C1 esterase inhibitors (C1-INH, Cinryze, Berinert), 66-67
CCI (corrected count increment) for platelets, 16-17, 160
Cell-washing devices, 180
Ceprotin (protein C concentrate), *56,* 65
Chagas disease, 242, 246
Check-group sample in massive transfusion, 206
Children. *See* Pediatric transfusion practices
Cinryze (C1 esterase inhibitors), 66-67
Circulatory overload, transfusion-associated, *228,* 233-234

Citrate-phosphate-dextrose (CPD)
Citrate-phosphate-dextrose-adenine (CPDA-1)
 red blood cells with, 2, 10, 11
 whole blood with, 5
Citrate-phosphate-dextrose-dextrose (CP2D), red blood cells with, 2
Citrate-related hypocalcemia due to therapeutic apheresis, 267
CJD (Creutzfeldt-Jakob disease), 246-247
Clopidogrel (Plavix)
 acquired platelet disorder due to, 116-117
 platelet function defect due to, 90-91
CMV. *See* Cytomegalovirus (CMV)
Coagadex (Factor X concentrate), *55,* 62, 105
Coagulation, disseminated intravascular, 14, 119
 due to acute hemolytic transfusion reaction, 223
Coagulation control proteins
 deficiency of, 124-125
 in hemostasis, 83-84
Coagulation factor inhibitors, direct-acting, 113-114
Coagulation monitoring, intraoperative, 183-184
Coagulopathy, and trauma, 120-121, 198
Cold-stored whole blood (cWB) in massive transfusion, 208
Colloid solutions, 69-70
Complement fixation in acute hemolytic transfusion reaction, 222

Conjugated estrogens, 122-123
Contact factor system in hemostasis, 84
Corifact (Factor XIII concentrate), 55, 66, 109
Corrected count increment (CCI) for platelets, 16-17, 160
CP2D (citrate-phosphate-dextrose-dextrose), 2
CPD (citrate-phosphate-dextrose), 2, 5, 10, 11
CPDA-1 (citrate-phosphate-dextrose-adenine)
CRASH-2 (Clinical Randomisation of an Antifibrinolytic in Significant Haemorrhage 2) trial, 210-211
Creutzfeldt-Jakob disease (CJD), 246-247
Crossmatching, 141-144, *143, 144*
  for intrauterine transfusion, 153
  for massive transfusion, 206-207
  platelet, 161
Crossmatch-to-transfusion (C:T) ratio, 178-179
Cryoprecipitated antihemophilic factor, *4,* 24-26
  for fibrinogen deficiency, 109
  for hemophilia A (Factor VIII deficiency), 98-99
  for von Willebrand disease, 96
Crystalloid solutions, 69-70
C:T (crossmatch-to-transfusion) ratio, 178-179
Cytapheresis, 258-263
Cytomegalovirus (CMV), 20, 245
  See also Leukocyte-reduced blood components

D

D antigen, prevention of alloimmunization to, 73-75
Dabigatran (Pradaxa), 114
Darbepoetin for anemia in premature infants, 155
DAT (direct antiglobulin test) for acute hemolytic transfusion reaction, 223
DDAVP. *See* Desmopressin (DDAVP, Stimate)
Delayed hemolytic transfusion reactions (DHTRs), 238-247
  air embolism as, 242
  etiology and pathogenesis of, 238-239
  extravascular, 239
  graft-vs-host disease as, 240-241
  hemosiderosis as, 241-242
  intravascular, 239
  posttransfusion purpura as, 240
  transfusion-transmitted diseases as, 242-247, *243*
Desmopressin (DDAVP, Stimate), 121
  for hemophilia A (Factor VIII deficiency), 98
  for massive transfusion, 211
  for platelet function defects, 90
  for von Willebrand disease, 92-95
Dextran, 69, 70, 174

DHTRs. *See* Delayed hemolytic transfusion reactions (DHTRs)
DIC (disseminated intravascular coagulation), 14, 119, 223
2,3-Diphosphoglycerate (2,3-DPG) in whole blood, 5
Direct antiglobulin test (DAT), 223
Direct-acting coagulation factor inhibitors, 113-114
Direct-acting oral anticoagulants (DOACs), 113-114
Directed oral anticoagulants, 113-114
Disseminated intravascular coagulation (DIC), 14, 119, 223
Drug-induced hemolysis, 230
Duffy system antigens, 239

E

EACA (epsilon aminocaproic acid), 121-122
Early trauma-induced coagulopathy (ETIC), 198
Ecchymosis, 85
ECP (extracorporeal photopheresis), 265
Edoxaban (Savaysa), 114
Effient (prasugrel)
    acquired platelet disorder due to, 116-117
    platelet function defect due to, 91
Eliquis (apixaban), 114
Eloctate (recombinant Factor VIII (rFVIII) Fc fusion protein), 59
Eltrombopag for platelet refractoriness, 161

Embolism, air, 242
EPO. *See* Erythropoietin (EPO)
Epoetin alfa, preoperative use of, 175
Epoetin beta, preoperative use of, 176
Epsilon aminocaproic acid (EACA), 121-122
Epstein-Barr virus, 246
Eptifibatide (Integrilin), acquired platelet disorder due to, 117
Erythrocytapheresis, 159, 262
Erythropoiesis-stimulating agents (ESAs), preoperative use of, 174-176
Erythropoietin (EPO), 155, 175-176
Estrogens, conjugated, 122-123
ETIC (early trauma-induced coagulopathy), 198
Exchange transfusion, 153-154
Exsanguination. *See* Massive transfusion
Extracorporeal photopheresis (ECP), 265
Extravascular hemolytic transfusion reactions, 223-225, *226*, 239

F

Factor II deficiency, 105
Factor V and Factor VIII deficiency, *108*
Factor V deficiency, 105, *106*
Factor VII deficiency, 105, *107*
Factor VIIa, recombinant (NovoSeven), *54,* 64
    for congenital Factor VII deficiency, 105

for management of inhibitors to Factor VIII or Factor IX, 103
for massive transfusion, 211
Factor VIII
  management of inhibitors to, 103-104
  recombinant porcine (Obizur), 59, 98
Factor VIII concentrates, 53-61, *54*, 98
Factor VIII deficiency, 92, 98-101, *100, 101*
Factor VIII products, extended half-life, 59-60
Factor IX, 102-104
Factor IX concentrates (Alprolix, Idelvion, REBINYN), *54,* 61-62, 102
Factor IX deficiency, 101-102
Factor X concentrate (Coagadex), *55,* 62, 105
Factor X deficiency, 105, *107*
Factor XI deficiency, 104, *107*
Factor XII deficiency, 109
Factor XIII assay, 87
Factor XIII concentrate (Corifact), *55,* 66, 109
Factor XIII deficiency, *107,* 109
Factor XIII subunit, recombinant (TRETTEN), 66, 109
Febrile nonhemolytic transfusion reaction (FNHTR), *227,* 231-232
FEIBA (activated prothrombin complex concentrates), *56,* 65, 103
Fetus, hemolytic disease of, 150-152

FFP (fresh frozen plasma), *4,* 20-21, 207
Fibrin, in hemostasis, 83, 84
Fibrin glue, 65-66
Fibrin sealant, 65-66
Fibrinogen assay, quantitative, 87
Fibrinogen concentrate (RiaSTAP), *54,* 65, 109, 211
Fibrinogen deficiency, *106,* 109
Fibrinolysis
  disorders of, 129-130
  evaluation of, 87
  in hemostasis, 84-85
Filter(s), 165
Filtered blood components. *See* Leukocyte-reduced blood components
Fixed-ratio component transfusion (FRCT) in massive hemorrhage, 200-201
FNHTR (febrile nonhemolytic transfusion reaction), *227,* 231-232
Fondaparinux (Arixtra), 112
Fresh frozen plasma (FFP), *4,* 20-21, 207
Frozen red cells, *3,* 34-35

G

Gamma globulin preparations, 70-71
Gamma irradiation, 30-31
G-CSF (granulocyte colony-stimulating factor), 18, 19
Gelatins, 69
Goal-directed component therapy (GDCT) in massive hemorrhage, 201-202
GPIIb/IIIa inhibitors, 91, 117

Graft-vs-host disease (GVHD), 240-241
  in hematopoietic progenitor cell transplantation, 146
  irradiated blood components for, 31
  in solid organ transplantation, 149
Granulocyte(s), *4,* 17-20
  contraindications and precautions for, 19-20
  description of, 17-18
  dose and administration of, 20
  indications for, 18-19
  for neonatal patients, 158
Granulocyte colony-stimulating factor (G-CSF), 18, 19
Group A plasma, low-titer group, in massive transfusion, 208
Group O uncrossmatched red cells for massive transfusion, 204-206
Group-specific blood components in massive transfusion, 206-207
GVHD. *See* Graft-vs-host disease

H

HAE (hereditary angioedema), 66-67
HBsAg (hepatitis B surface antigen), 242
HBV (hepatitis B virus), 242, 243, *243*
HCV (hepatitis C virus), 242, 243, *243*
HDFN (hemolytic disease of the fetus and newborn), 150-152
Hematopoietic progenitor cell (HPC) transplantation, 145-146, *147-148*
Hemodilution, acute normovolemic, 179
Hemoglobin monitoring, intraoperative, 184
Hemoglobin thresholds, 156, 185
Hemoglobinuria in acute hemolytic transfusion reaction, 222
Hemolysis, 230-231
Hemolytic disease of the fetus and newborn (HDFN), 150-152
Hemolytic transfusion reactions (HTRs), 221
  acute, 221-225
    clinical presentation of, 223-225
    diagnosis of, 222-223
    drug-induced, 230
    etiology and pathogenesis of, 222-223
    extravascular, 223-225, *226*
    intravascular, 222, *224, 226*
    nonimmune, 231
    severity of, 223
    sickle cell, 225-230
    workup for, 223-225, *224-225*
  delayed, 238-247
    air embolism as, 242
    etiology and pathogenesis of, 238-239

extravascular, 239
graft-vs-host disease as, 240-241
hemosiderosis as, 241-242
intravascular, 239
posttransfusion purpura as, 240
transfusion-transmitted diseases as, 242-247, *243*
Hemolytic-uremic syndrome (HUS), 128, 264
Hemophilia A, 98-101, *100, 101*
Hemophilia B, 101-102
Hemorrhage, 203-204, 209
See also Massive transfusion
Hemosiderosis, 241-242
Hemostasis
  blood vessels in, 81-82
  coagulation proteins in, 83-84
  defined, 81
  natural anticoagulant systems and fibrinolysis in, 84-85
  overview of, 81-85
  platelets in, 82-83
  stages of, 81
Hemostatic agents, topical, 123
Hemostatic disorders, 81-113
  acquired, 110-121
    due to antiplatelet agents, 116-117
    coagulopathy of trauma and massive tissue injury as, 120-121
    disseminated intravascular coagulation as, 119
    due to heparins and directed oral anticoagulants, 111-115
    due to liver disease, 117-118
    management in patients on anticoagulant drugs of, 115-116
    vitamin K deficiency and vitamin K antagonists as, 110-111
  congenital, 91-110
    alpha$_2$-plasmin inhibitor deficiency as, 109-110
    Factor V and Factor VIII deficiency as, *108*
    Factor V deficiency, 105, *106*
    Factor VII deficiency, 105, *107*
    Factor X deficiency, *107*
    Factor XI deficiency, 104, *107*
    Factor XII deficiency, 109
    Factor XIII deficiency, *107,* 109
    fibrinogen deficiency, *106,* 109
    hemophilia A (Factor VIII deficiency), 98-101, *100, 101*
    hemophilia B (Factor IX deficiency), 101-102
    management of inhibitors to Factor VIII or Factor IX, 103-104
    non-vitamin-K-dependent Factor V deficiency, 105, *106*
    other, 105-109, *106-108*
    prothrombin deficiency, *106*

281

vitamin-K-dependent factor deficiencies, 105, *108*
von Willebrand disease, 91-98, *93-94, 97, 100*
disorders of fibrinolysis, 129-130
evaluation of, 85-88
platelet disorders as, 88-91
  due to platelet function defects, 90-91
  thrombocytopenia as, 88-89
prohemostatic drugs for, 121-123
thrombotic disorders as, 123-129
  antiphospholipid syndrome as, 125-126
  due to deficiency of coagulation control proteins, 124-125
  heparin-induced thrombocytopenia as, 126-127
  thrombotic microangiopathies as, 127-129
Hemostatic resuscitation in trauma and massive bleeding. *See* Massive transfusion
Hemovigilance, 247
Heparin(s), 111-112
Heparin-induced thrombocytopenia (HIT), 14, 126-127
Hepatitis, 242, 243, *243*
Hepatitis B surface antigen (HBsAg), 242
Hepatitis B virus (HBV), 242, 243, *243*
Hepatitis C virus (HCV), 242, 243, *243*
Hepatitis E virus (HEV), 243
Hereditary angioedema (HAE), 66-67
HES (hydroxyethyl starch), 69, 70
HGA (human granulocytic anaplasmosis), 246
High-molecular-weight (HMW) dextran, iron supplementation with, 174
HIT (heparin-induced thrombocytopenia), 14, 126-127
HIV (human immunodeficiency virus), 242, *243*, 244
HLA antibodies in platelet refractoriness, 160-161
HPC (hematopoietic progenitor cell) transplantation, 145-146, *147-148*
HTLVs (human T-cell lymphotropic viruses), 242, 245
HTRs. *See* Hemolytic transfusion reactions (HTRs)
Human granulocytic anaplasmosis (HGA), 246
Human herpesvirus 8, 246
Human immunodeficiency virus (HIV), 242, *243*, 244
Human T-cell lymphotropic viruses (HTLVs), 242, 245
Human-plasma-derived Factor VIII concentrate, 58
Humate-P (von Willebrand factor-containing Factor VIII concentrate), 59
  for von Willebrand disease, 95-97, *97, 100*

HUS (hemolytic-uremic syndrome), 128, 264
Hydroxyethyl starch (HES), 69, 70
Hyperimmune globulin preparations, 70-71
Hypocalcemia, citrate-related, due to therapeutic apheresis, 267
Hypotension, transfusion-associated, 223, *229,* 235-236

I

Idelvion (Factor IX concentrates), *54,* 61-62, 102
Identification of blood components, 162
Idiopathic thrombocytopenic purpura (ITP), 14, 154-155
IMIG (intramuscular immune globulin), 71
Immune acute transfusion reaction, *224, 226*
Immune globulins, *57,* 70-72
 See also Rh Immune Globulin
Immune thrombocytopenia (ITP), 14, 154-155
Infusion devices, 163-164
Integrilin (eptifibatide), acquired platelet disorder due to, 117
Intramuscular immune globulin (IMIG), 71
Intraoperative blood recovery, 179-180
Intrauterine transfusion, 152-153
Intravascular hemolytic transfusion reactions
 acute, 222, *224, 226*
 delayed, 239
Intravenous immune globulin (IVIG), 71, 72, 155
Intravenous solutions, concomitant use of, 164
Iron supplementation, preoperative, 173-174
Irradiated blood components, 30-33
 contraindications and precautions for, 31
 description of, 30-31
 dosage and administration of, 33
 indications for, 31, *32*
ITP (idiopathic thrombocytopenic purpura), 14, 154-155
IVIG (intravenous immune globulin), 71, 72, 155

K

Kcentra. *See* Prothrombin complex concentrates
Kell system antigens
 antibodies to, 150
 delayed hemolytic transfusion reaction due to, 239
Kidd system antigens, delayed hemolytic transfusion reaction due to, 239

L

Lactate dehydrogenase (LDH) in acute hemolytic transfusion reaction, 223
Lactated Ringer's solution, 69
LDL (low-density lipoprotein) removal, 264-265

Leukocytapheresis, 262
Leukocyte reduction filters, 165
Leukocyte-reduced blood components, 26-30
  contraindications and precautions for, 30
  description of, 26-28
  dose and administration of, 30
  indications for, 28-30
  methods for producing, 27-28
  platelets, *3,* 27
  red cells, *2,* 27
Lipid apheresis, 264-265
Lipid removal, selective, 264-265
Liquid plasma in massive transfusion, 207-208
Liver disease, acquired platelet disorder in, 117-118
Low-density lipoprotein (LDL) removal, 264-265
Low-molecular-weight heparin (LMWH), 112
Low-titer group A plasma in massive transfusion, 208
Lupus anticoagulant, 125-126
Lysine analogues, synthetic, 121-122

M

Malaria, 246
Massive tissue injury, coagulopathy of, 120-121
Massive transfusion, 197-199
Massive transfusion protocol (MTP), 199-211
  adjunctive therapies in, 210-211
  blood component transfusion strategies in, 200-202
  cold-stored whole blood in, 208
  defined, 199
  group O uncrossmatched RBCs in, 204-206
  indications for, 199
  location of, 199
  major components of, 202
  MTP packages for, 204
  for obstetric hemorrhage, 209
  operational aspects of, 202-210
  overview of, 199-200
  performance improvement monitoring for, 209-210
  RhD-positive components in RhD-negative or RhD-status-unknown patients, 207
  sample algorithm for, *203*
  thawed plasma, liquid plasma, and low-titer group A plasma in, 207-208
  transition to group-specific blood components in, 206-207
  when to activate, 202-204, *205*
Massive transfusion protocol (MTP) packages, 204
Maximum surgical blood order schedule (MSBOS), 177-179
Medications with blood transfusion, 164
Metabolic complications, 238
Microaggregate blood filters, 165

Microangiopathies, thrombotic, 127-129, 264
MSBOS (maximum surgical blood order schedule), 177-179
MTP. *See* Massive transfusion protocol

N

Neonatal alloimmune thrombocytopenia (NAIT), 154-155
Neonatal thrombocytopenia, 154-155
Neonatal transfusion practices, 153-158
Neuromyelitis optica (NMO), 264
Newborn, hemolytic disease of, 150-152
Non-ABO red cell antibodies, acute hemolytic transfusion reaction due to, 222
Nonimmune hemolysis, 231
Normal saline, 69, 164
NovoSeven. *See* Factor VIIa, recombinant (NovoSeven)

O

Obizur (recombinant porcine Factor VIII), 59
 for hemophilia A (Factor VIII deficiency), 98
 for management of inhibitors to Factor VIII, 59
Obstetric hemorrhage, 203-204, 209
Obstetric shock index, 203-204
Obstetric transfusion practices, 150-153

Octaplas, 21, 22, 36, 37, 38
Oral contraceptives, 122-123
Oxygen therapeutics, 35-36

P

PAD (preoperative autologous blood donation), 176-177
PAI-1 (plasminogen activator inhibitor) in hemostasis, 85
Parasite-related disease, 246
Parvovirus B19, 245-246
PAS (platelet additive solution), *3,* 12-13
Pathogen inactivation, 36-38
Patient blood management (PBM), 171-187
 blood utilization review for, 186-187
 concept of, 171
 nonsurgical/preoperative issues for, 172-177
  evaluating anemia as, 172-173
  iron supplementation as, 173-174
  preoperative autologous blood donation as, 176-177
  preoperative use of erythropoiesis-stimulating agents as, 174-176
 perioperative techniques for, 177-184
  acute normovolemic hemodilution as, 179
  intraoperative blood recovery as, 179-180
  other coagulation monitoring as, 183-184

point-of-care testing as, 180-181
surgical blood order schedule as, 177-179
viscoelastic coagulation monitoring as, 181-183, *182*
postoperative, 184-185
postoperative blood recovery as, 184-185
prevention of excessive iatrogenic blood loss as, 184
transfusion thresholds as, 185
program structure for, 171-172
PBM. *See* Patient blood management (PBM)
PCCs. *See* Prothrombin complex concentrates
Pediatric transfusion practices, 158-159, 197-198
Percutaneous umbilical blood sampling (PUBS), 152
Perioperative techniques
acute normovolemic hemodilution, 179
intraoperative blood recovery as, 179-180
other coagulation monitoring as, 183-184
for patient blood management, 177-184
point-of-care testing as, 180-181
surgical blood order schedule as, 177-179
viscoelastic coagulation monitoring as, 181-183, *182*
Petechiae, 85

PF24 (Plasma Frozen Within 24 Hours After Phlebotomy), *4*, 21, 207
PFA-100 (platelet function analyzer), 86
Photopheresis, extracorporeal, 265
Plasma, *4*, 20-24
contraindications and precautions for, 22-23
description of, 20-21
dosage and administration of, 23-24
for Factor V deficiency, 105
fresh frozen, *4*, 20-21, 207
indications for, 21-22
liquid, in massive transfusion, 207-208
low-titer group A, in massive transfusion, 208
in massive transfusion, 207-208
for neonatal patients, 157
pathogen-reduced, 21
storage and shelf life of, 21
thawed, *4*, 21, 207
for vitamin-K-dependent factor deficiency, 105
Plasma Cryoprecipitate Reduced, 22
Plasma derivatives, 53-75, *54-57*
albumin, *57*, 67-68
antithrombin concentrate, *56*, 63-64
C1 esterase inhibitors, 66-67
Factor VIIa (recombinant), *54*, 64
Factor VIII concentrates, 53-61, *54*

Factor IX concentrates, *54,* 61-62
Factor X concentrate, *55,* 62
Factor XIII concentrate, *55,* 66
fibrin sealant, 65-66
fibrinogen concentrate, *54,* 65
immune globulins, *57,* 70-72
plasma protein fraction, *57,* 67-68
protein C concentrate, *56,* 65
prothrombin complex concentrate, *55, 56,* 62-63
Rh Immune Globulin, *57,* 72-75
synthetic volume expanders as, 69-70
Plasma discoloration in acute hemolytic transfusion reaction, 222
Plasma exchange, therapeutic, 263-264
Plasma frozen within 24 hours after phlebotomy (PF24), *4,* 21, 207
Plasma protein fraction (PPF), *57,* 67-68
Plasmalyte with blood transfusion, 164
Plasmapheresis, 263
Plasmin in hemostasis, 84-85
Plasminogen activator inhibitor (PAI-1) in hemostasis, 85
Plasmodium falciparum, 246
Platelet(s)
  apheresis, *3,* 12, 16
  corrected count increment (CCI) for, 16-17
  defined, 82
  in hemostasis, 82-83
  leukocyte reduced, *3,* 27
  random-donor. *See* Platelet components
  storage and shelf life of, 12
Platelet additive solution (PAS), *3,* 12-13
Platelet components, *3,* 12-17
  ABO-incompatible, 15, 17
  bacterial contamination of, 14
  composition of, *3*
  contraindications and precautions for, 14-15
  description of, 12-13
  dose and administration of, 15-17
  indications for, *3,* 13-14
  pathogen inactivation of, *13*
  red cells in, 15
  volume of, *3,* 12
Platelet concentrates. *See* Platelet components
Platelet count, 86
Platelet crossmatching, 161
Platelet disorders, 88-91
Platelet function analyzer (PFA-100), 86
Platelet function defects, 90-91
Platelet function studies, intraoperative, 183
Platelet refractoriness, management of, 159-161
Platelet transfusions, 88-89, 157-158
Plateletpheresis, 262-263
Plavix (clopidogrel)
  acquired platelet disorder due to, 116-117
  platelet function defect due to, 90-91

Point-of-care testing (POCT), 180-181
Porcine factor, recombinant (Obizur), 59, 98, 104
Postoperative blood management, 184-185
Postpartum hemorrhage (PPH), 203-204, 209
Posttransfusion purpura (PTP), 240
PPF (plasma protein fraction), *57,* 67-68
Pradaxa (dabigatran), 114
Pragmatic Randomized Optimal Platelet and Plasma Ratios (PROPPR) study, 200-201
Prasugrel (Effient), 91, 116-117
Premature infants, anemia in, 155
Preoperative autologous blood donation (PAD), 176-177
Preoperative blood management issues, 172-177
  autologous blood donation as, 176-177
  evaluating anemia as, 172-173
  iron supplementation as, 173-174
  use of erythropoiesis-stimulating agents as, 174-176
Prions, 246-247
Profilnine SD. *See* Prothrombin complex concentrates
Prohemostatic drugs, 121-123
PROPPR (Pragmatic Randomized Optimal Platelet and Plasma Ratios) study, 200-201

Prospective, Observational, Multicenter, Major Trauma Transfusion (PROMTT) study, 200
Protease inhibitors in hemostasis, 84
Protein C, in hemostasis, 84
Protein C concentrate (Ceprotin), *56,* 65
Protein C deficiency, 125
Protein S deficiency, 125
Prothrombin complex concentrates, *55,* 62-63
  activated, *56,* 65
  for management of bleeding in patients on anticoagulant drugs, 115-116
  in massive transfusion, 211
  for vitamin-K-dependent factor deficiency, 105
Prothrombin deficiency, *106*
Prothrombin time (PT), 86, 87
Prothrombin time/international normalized ratio (PT/INR), 183
PTP (posttransfusion purpura), 240
PUBS (percutaneous umbilical blood sampling), 152
Purpura
  idiopathic thrombocytopenic, 14, 154-155
  posttransfusion, 240
  thrombotic thrombocytopenic, 14, 264

R

Rapid infusion systems, 164
RBCs. *See* Red Blood Cell(s)

REBINYN (Factor IX concentrates), *54,* 61-62
  for hemophilia B (Factor IX deficiency), 102
Recombinant Factor VIIa (NovoSeven), *54,* 64
  for congenital Factor VII deficiency, 105
  for management of inhibitors to Factor VIII or Factor IX, 103
  in massive transfusion, 211
Recombinant Factor VIII (rFVIII), 58-59, 98
Recombinant Factor VIII (rFVIII) Fc fusion protein (Eloctate), 59
Recombinant Factor VIII (rFVIII) PEGylated (Adynovate), 59
Recombinant Factor VIII (rFVIII) single chain (Afstyla), 59
Recombinant Factor IX for hemophilia B (Factor IX deficiency), 102
Recombinant Factor XIII subunit (TRETTEN), 66, 109
Recombinant human erythropoietin (rHuEPO), 155, 175-176
Red Blood Cell(s) (RBCs)
  with additive solution, *2,* 10, 11
  apheresis, *2*
  composition of, *2*
  contraindications and precautions for, 10-11
  deglycerolized, *3*
  description of, 9-10
  dosage and administration of, 11
  frozen, *3,* 34-35
  indications for, *2,* 10
  leukocyte reduced, *2,* 27
  for neonatal patients, 156-157, 158
  storage and shelf life of, *6-7,* 10
  volume of, *2*
  washed, *2,* 33-34
Red Blood Cell (RBC) units/patient, 178-179
Red cell components. *See* Red Blood Cells
Red cell substitutes, 35-36
ReoPro (abciximab), acquired platelet disorder due to, 117
rFVIII (recombinant Factor VIII) Fc fusion protein, 59
rFVIII (recombinant Factor VIII) PEGylated, 59
rFVIII (recombinant Factor VIII) single chain, 59
Rh antigens, delayed hemolytic transfusion reaction due to, 239
Rh factor, 15
Rh Immune Globulin, *57,* 72-75
  antepartum, 73-74, 151
  description of, 72-73
  postpartum, 74-75, 151
  special considerations for, 75
RhD antigen, antibody to, 150, 151
RhD-positive components in massive transfusion, 207
RhoGAM. *See* Rh Immune Globulin

Rhophylac. *See* Rh Immune Globulin
rHuEPO (recombinant human erythropoietin), 155, 175-176
RiaSTAP (fibrinogen concentrate), *54,* 65, 109
    in massive transfusion, 211
Rivaroxaban (Xarelto), 114
Romiplostim for platelet refractoriness, 161
Rotational thromboelastometry (ROTEM), 87-88
    intraoperative, 181-183, *182*
    for massive transfusion, 201

S

Savaysa (edoxaban), 114
Selective lipid removal, 264-265
Shock due to acute hemolytic transfusion reaction, 223
Sickle cell disease, 158-159
Sickle cell hemolytic transfusion reaction syndrome, 225-230
Sodium chloride hypotonic solution, 69
Solid organ transplantation, 146-149
Solvent/detergent treatment for pathogen inactivation, 36-38
Standard surgical blood order schedule (SSBOS), 177-179
Stimate. *See* Desmopressin (DDAVP, Stimate)
Surgical blood order schedule, 177-179
Surgical blood ordering practices, 141-144, *143, 144*
Synthetic lysine analogues, 121-122
Synthetic volume expanders, 69-70
Syphilis, 242

T

TACO (transfusion-associated circulatory overload), *228,* 233-234
TAFI (thrombin-activatable fibrinolysis inhibitor) in hemostasis, 83
TA-GVHD. *See* Transfusion-associated graft-vs-host disease (TA-GVHD)
TASH (trauma-associated severe hemorrhage) score, 202, *205*
T/C (type and crossmatch), 141-144, *143, 144*
T-cell inactivation for neonatal transfusions, 158
TEG. *See* Thromboelastography
TF (tissue factor) in hemostasis, 82, 83
TFPI (tissue factor pathway inhibitor) in hemostasis, 83
Thalassemia syndromes, 159
Thawed plasma in massive transfusion, 207
Therapeutic apheresis, 257-268
    complications of, 266-268
    defined, 257
    forms of, 258-265
        cytapheresis as, 258-263
        extracorporeal photopheresis as, 265
        selective lipid removal (lipid apheresis) as, 264-265

therapeutic plasma exchanges as, 263-264
indications for, 257-258, *258-261*
procedural considerations with, 265-266
Therapeutic cytapheresis, 258-263
Therapeutic plasma exchange (TPE), 263-264
Thermal effects, acute transfusion reactions due to, 237-238
Thienopyridines, 90-91, 116-117
Thrombin, in hemostasis, 83
Thrombin generation assays, 87
Thrombin inhibitors, direct-acting, 113-114
Thrombin time (TT), 87
Thrombin-activatable fibrinolysis inhibitor (TAFI) in hemostasis, 83
Thrombocytopenia, 88-89
  heparin-induced, 14, 126-127
  immune, 14, 154-155
  neonatal, 154-155
Thromboelastography (TEG), 87-88
  intraoperative, 181-183, *182*
  for massive transfusion, 201
Thromboembolism, 123
Thrombophilia, 123-124
Thrombopoietin receptor agonists for platelet refractoriness, 161
Thrombotic disorders, 123-129
  antiphospholipid syndrome as, 125-126
  due to deficiency of coagulation control proteins, 124-125
  heparin-induced thrombocytopenia as, 126-127
  thrombotic microangiopathies as, 127-129
Thrombotic microangiopathies (TMAs), 127-129, 264
Thrombotic thrombocytopenic purpura (TTP), 14, 264
Ticagrelor, platelet function defect due to, 91
Tirofiban (Aggrastat), acquired platelet disorder due to, 117
Tissue factor (TF) in hemostasis, 82, 83
Tissue factor pathway inhibitor (TFPI) in hemostasis, 83
Tissue plasminogen activator (tPA) in hemostasis, 84-85
TMAs (thrombotic microangiopathies), 127-129, 264
Topical hemostatic agents, 123
TPE (therapeutic plasma exchange), 263-264
TRALI (transfusion-related acute lung injury), *228,* 234-235
Tranexamic acid, 121-122, 210-211
Transfusion index, 178-179
Transfusion practices, 141-165
  for blood administration, 161-165
    blood component identification as, 161-162
    blood warming as, 163

291

with concomitant use of
intravenous solutions,
164
filters in, 165
infusion devices in, 163-
164
time limits for infusing
blood components as,
162
for hematopoietic progenitor
cell transplantation, 145-
146, *147-148*
for management of platelet
refractoriness, 159-161
neonatal, 153-158
for exchange transfusion,
153-154
for neonatal
thrombocytopenia, 154-
155
for routine transfusion,
155-158
obstetric, 150-153
for hemolytic disease of
the fetus and newborn,
150-152
for intrauterine
transfusion, 152-153
pediatric, 158-159
for solid organ
transplantation, 146-149
for surgical blood ordering,
141-144, *143, 144*
for urgent transfusion, 144-
145
Transfusion reactions, 221-247
acute, 221-238, *226-229*
allergic, *227,* 232-233
due to bacterial
contamination, *224-
225, 229,* 236-237
defined, 221
drug-induced hemolysis
as, 230
extravascular hemolytic,
223-225, *226*
febrile nonhemolytic,
227, 231-232
hemolytic, 221-225
hypotension as, *229,* 235-
236
immune, *224, 226*
intravascular hemolytic,
222, *224, 226*
metabolic, 238
nonimmune hemolysis as,
231
sickle cell hemolytic,
225-230
due to thermal effects,
237-238
transfusion-associated
circulatory overload
(TACO) as, *228,* 233-
234
transfusion-related acute
lung injury (TRALI) as,
228, 234-235
workup of, *224-225*
delayed, 238-247
air embolism as, 242
etiology and pathogenesis
of, 238-239
extravascular, 239
graft-vs-host disease as,
240-241
hemosiderosis as, 241-242
intravascular, 239

posttransfusion purpura as, 240
transfusion-transmitted diseases as, 242-247, *243*
hemolytic, 221
acute, 221-225
air embolism, 242
delayed, 238-247
drug-induced, 230
extravascular, 223-225, *226*
graft-vs-host disease, 240-241
hemosiderosis, 241-242
intravascular, 222, *224, 226*
nonimmune, 231
posttransfusion purpura, 240
sickle cell, 225-230
transfusion-transmitted diseases, 242-247, *243*
hemovigilance for, 247
Transfusion thresholds, 156, 185
Transfusion-associated circulatory overload (TACO), *228,* 233-234
Transfusion-associated graft-vs-host disease (TA-GVHD), 240-241
in hematopoietic progenitor cell transplantation, 146
irradiated blood components for, 31
in solid organ transplantation, 149
Transfusion-related acute lung injury (TRALI), *228,* 234-235
Transfusion-transmitted diseases, 242-247
cytomegalovirus, 245
Epstein-Barr virus, 246
hepatitis, 242, 243, *243*
HIV, 242, *243,* 244
HTLVs, 242, 245
human herpesvirus 8, 246
parasite-related, 246
parvovirus B19 as, 245-246
due to prions, 246-247
residual risk of, 242, *243*
screening of blood donations for, 242
West Nile virus, 242, 244
Zika virus, 242, 244-245
Transplantation
hematopoietic progenitor cell (HPC), 145-146, *147-148*
solid organ, 146-149
Trauma
coagulopathy of, 120-121
See also Massive transfusion
Trauma-associated severe hemorrhage (TASH) score, 202, *205*
Trauma-induced coagulopathy, early, 198
TRETTEN (Factor XIII subunit, recombinant), 66, 109
Trypanosoma cruzi, 242, 246
TT (thrombin time), 87
TTP (thrombotic thrombocytopenic purpura), 14, 264
Type and crossmatch (T/C), 141-144, *143, 144*
Type and screen (T/S), 141

U

Umbilical blood sampling, percutaneous, 152

Uncrossmatched red blood cells for massive transfusion, 204-206
Unfractionated heparin (UFH), 111-112
Urgent transfusion, 144-145

V

Variant Creutzfeldt-Jakob disease (vCJD), 246-247
Venous thromboembolic (VTE) disease, 123-124
Viscoelastic coagulation monitoring, 181-183, *182*
Viscoelastic testing, 87-88
intraoperative, 181-183, *182*
for massive transfusion, 201
Vitamin K antagonists, 110-111
Vitamin K deficiency, 110-111
Vitamin-K-dependent factor deficiencies, 105, *108*
Volume expanders, synthetic, 69-70
von Willebrand disease (vWD), 91-98
classification of, 92, *93-94*
clinical manifestations of, 92
defined, 91-92
diagnosis of, 92
treatment of, 92-98, *93-95, 97, 100*
von Willebrand factor (vWF), 91-97
von Willebrand factor (vWF) concentrate (VONVENDI), 59
von Willebrand factor (vWF)-containing Factor VIII concentrates (Humate-P, Alphanate, Wilate), 59
for von Willebrand disease, 95-97, *97, 100*
VTE (venous thromboembolic) disease, 123-124
vWD. *See* von Willebrand disease (vWD)
vWF. *See* von Willebrand factor (vWF)

W

Warfarin, 110-111
Washed blood components, *2,* 33-34
WBIT (wrong blood in tube) miscollections in massive transfusion, 206
West Nile virus (WNV), 242, 244
Whole blood (WB), 5-9
cold-stored, in massive transfusion, 208
composition of, *2, 5*
contraindications and precautions for, 8-9
description of, 5
dosage and administration of, 9
hematocrit of, 5
indications for, *2,* 8
processing into components of, 1
storage and shelf life of, 5, *6-7*
volume of, *2,* 5
Whole blood viscoelastic monitoring, 87-88
Wilate (von Willebrand factor-containing Factor VIII concentrate), 59, 95-97, *97, 100*

WinRho SDF. *See* Rh Immune Globulin
WNV (West Nile virus), 242, 244
Wrong blood in tube (WBIT) miscollections in massive transfusion, 206

X-Z

Xarelto (rivaroxaban), 114
X-ray irradiation, 31
Zika virus (ZIKV), 242, 244-245